www.harcourt-international.com

Bringing you products from all Harcourt Health Sciences companies including Baillière Tindall, Churchill Livingstone, Mosby and W.B. Saunders

- ▶ **Browse** for latest information on new books, journals and electronic products

- ▶ **Search** for information on over 20 000 published titles with full product information including tables of contents and sample chapters

- ▶ **Keep up to date** with our extensive publishing programme in your field by registering with **eAlert** or requesting postal updates

- ▶ **Secure online ordering** with prompt delivery, as well as full contact details to order by phone, fax or post

- ▶ **News** of special features and promotions

If you are based in the following countries, please visit the country-specific site to receive full details of product availability and local ordering information

USA: www.harcourthealth.com

Canada: www.harcourtcanada.

Australia: www.harcourt.com.a

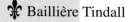 Baillière Tindall   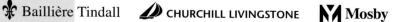 CHURCHILL LIVINGSTONE   Mosby   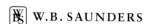 W.B. SAUNDERS

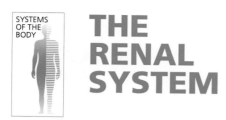

THE
RENAL
SYSTEM

SYSTEMS OF THE BODY

SYSTEMS
OF THE
BODY

Commissioning Editor: Michael Parkinson
Project Development Manager: Lynn Watt
Project Controller: Frances Affleck
Designer: Erik Bigland

THE RENAL SYSTEM

Michael J. Field MD, BS, BSc(Hons), FRACP
Professor of Medicine, Concord Hospital, Concord, NSW, Australia

Carol A. Pollock MB, BS, PhD, FRACP
Professor of Medicine, Royal North Shore Hospital, St Leonards, NSW, Australia

David C. Harris MD, BS, FRACP
Associate Professor of Medicine, Westmead Hospital, Westmead, NSW, Australia

All of Department of Medicine, University of Sydney, Australia

Illustrations by Robert Britton

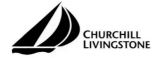
CHURCHILL
LIVINGSTONE

EDINBURGH LONDON NEW YORK PHILADELPHIA ST LOUIS SYDNEY TORONTO 2001

CHURCHILL LIVINGSTONE
An imprint of Harcourt Publishers Limited

© Harcourt Publishers Limited 2001

◢ is a registered trademark of Harcourt Publishers Limited

The right of Michael J. Field, Carol A. Pollock and David C. Harris
to be identified as authors of this work has been asserted by them
in accordance with the Copyright, Designs and Patents Act 1988.

First published 2001

ISBN 0–443–06478–4

British Library Cataloguing in Publication Data
A catalogue record for this book is available from the British
Library

Library of Congress Cataloging in Publication Data
A catalog record for this book is available from the Library of
Congress

Note
Medical knowledge is constantly changing. As new information
becomes available, changes in treatment, procedures, equipment
and the use of drugs become necessary. The editors/authors/
contributors and the publishers have, as far as it is possible, taken
care to ensure that the information given in this text is accurate
and up to date. However, readers are strongly advised to confirm
that the information, especially with regard to drug usage,
complies with the latest legislation and standards of practice.

The
Publisher's
policy is to use
**paper manufactured
from sustainable forests**

Printed in Spain

II

Medical students, and indeed many practising doctors, have generally regarded learning about the normal kidney and its diseases as one of the more difficult areas in medicine. Many of the underlying concepts of normal structure and function may seem rather abstract, and the classification and manifestations of disease states can be confusing.

One of the reasons for this perceived difficulty in studying the kidney may be that the component disciplines have traditionally been presented largely in isolation from each other, so that the relationships between normal and abnormal structure and function, and the relevance of basic scientific descriptions to clinical problems, has not been made clear.

This book, like others in the Systems of the Body series, aims to guide beginning medical students in learning about the kidney by adopting a closely integrated approach. Each chapter is based around a clinical case scenario, and the process of working through the patient's problems leads to exploration of a variety of relevant material, drawn from the basic and clinical sciences as required. For example, in the first chapter, the presentation of a child with a probable urinary infection leads to consideration of the normal anatomy of the urinary tract and of developmental abnormalities which may predispose to urinary infection. At the same time, aspects of microbiology, antibiotic pharmacology, and modalities for imaging the urinary tract are dealt with, in context.

By this means, most of the important basic sciences relevant to understanding the structure, function and diseases of the renal system are covered, at a level appropriate to medical students in the first part of their course. The approach taken complements the philosophy of problem-based learning (PBL), which is being adopted by ever increasing numbers of medical schools throughout the world, though it should be equally useful to students enrolled in more conventional programs. Indeed, the book should in no way be seen as short-circuiting the process of self-directed learning which is at the heart of PBL-based courses, and it is expected that students will also consult conventional discipline-based textbooks and the medical literature to expand the horizons of their understanding of the subject-matter of the book.

In order to acknowledge that many students using this text will have had little clinical experience at this early stage of their course, we have provided a Glossary to define unfamiliar clinical terms used in the book (other than words which are explained within the context of the relevant chapter). Such terms are shown in bold in the text on their first occurrence. Each chapter ends with some self-assessment exercises (a case study and some short answer questions) designed to promote reflection on the main issues raised in the chapter, and full answers are provided at the end of the book.

While there are many developments in basic renal science, and many clinical conditions involving the kidney, which are not covered in this introductory book, we feel confident that students who master the material we have included here will be in a good position to take the study of the kidney further in their later undergraduate and postgraduate training.

It is a pleasure to acknowledge the enthusiasm and assistance of the publishers in producing this volume in the Systems of the Body series. In particular, the vision and leadership of Michael Parkinson, Commissioning Editor, and the attention to detail of Sarah Keer-Keer and Lynn Watt, Project Development Managers, were greatly appreciated.

A number of our colleagues assisted by offering suggestions for the improvement of the text, or by providing material for the illustrations. Dr George Kotsiou, of the Royal North Shore Hospital, Sydney, contributed to the microbiology sections of Chapter 1, while various photographic images were provided by colleagues at Concord Hospital, Westmead Hospital, Royal North Shore Hospital and the Department of Pathology, University of Sydney.

A special word of thanks is due to Beverley Smith, who assisted with preparation of the manuscript, and, as is traditional (but also appropriate), we would all like to acknowledge the patience shown by our families during the period in which this book was being written.

CONTENTS

GLOMERULONEPHRITIS AND THE ACUTE NEPHRITIC SYNDROME 87

DIABETIC NEPHROPATHY AND CHRONIC RENAL FAILURE 97

HYPERTENSION AND THE KIDNEY 107

URINARY TRACT OBSTRUCTION AND STONES 121

DRUGS AND THE KIDNEY 131

URINARY TRACT STRUCTURE AND INFECTION

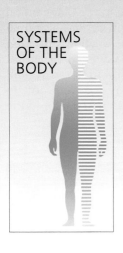

SYSTEMS
OF THE
BODY

Chapter objectives

After studying this chapter you should be able to:

① Describe the structure and embryological origins of the major anatomical components of the urinary tract, namely kidneys, ureters, bladder and urethra.

② Understand the clinical distinction between upper and lower urinary tract infections.

③ Describe the organisms commonly associated with urinary infections and the mechanisms which make these organisms uropathogenic.

④ Describe the underlying factors associated with complicated urinary tract infections.

⑤ Select the most appropriate imaging techniques for the urinary tract when structural abnormalities are suspected.

⑥ Understand the principles of treatment of upper and lower urinary tract infections.

⑦ Describe the anatomical abnormalities and complications occurring in patients with vesicoureteric reflux.

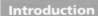

Introduction

The kidneys are highly specialized organs that function to regulate the volume and chemical composition of the body fluids. In carrying out this function, they excrete most water-soluble waste products in urine. Once the urine is formed, it is collected and stored in the bladder. The bladder then empties intermittently during the process known as micturition.

When the normal processes of embryological development are disturbed, defects may develop in the structure of the urinary tract that interfere with the normal production and flow of urine. As a consequence, urinary tract infection may occur, and may be the initial clue that a structural abnormality of the urinary tract exists. This chapter, illustrated by the case of such an infection in a child, will introduce the basic structure and development of the kidneys and urinary tract, and discuss the common problem of urinary tract infection.

Urinary tract structure and infection box 1

A febrile child

Tommy Baron is a 2-year-old boy who presents with a fever up to 39°C of 24 h duration. Although initially complaining of abdominal pain and unable to be comforted, he is now clearly ill, with lethargy and diffuse abdominal tenderness. His blood pressure is normal at 70/40 mmHg. Examination is otherwise unremarkable. **Urinalysis** shows blood +++, protein ++ and is positive for leucocyte esterase (markers of white cells) and nitrites (markers of bacterial action).

We can infer from this information that Tommy is systemically unwell, with infection being the likely problem. The urinary abnormalities suggest the urinary tract is a source of the sepsis.

To understand the structural basis of this illness, we should initially familiarize ourselves with the anatomical components of the urinary tract. We can then consider whether Tommy is likely to have any abnormality that may predispose him to infection.

Normal anatomy of the urinary tract

The urinary tract is made up of the kidneys, ureters, bladder and urethra (Fig. 1.1). The kidneys are normally considered to be the upper urinary tract, whereas the remaining structures may be considered to be the lower urinary tract. There are normally two kidneys, each placed retroperitoneally in the posterior abdominal wall on either side of the spine at the level

of the upper lumbar vertebrae. Each kidney is 10–14 cm in length in adults and is surrounded by a fibrous capsule within perirenal fat. The renal hilus on the concave medial aspect of the kidney is the point of entry for the arteries, veins and nerves, and exit for the urine drainage system. The urine formed by the kidney initially drains into the renal pelvis, which may be considered as the dilated portion of the ureter which links the kidney to the bladder. The urine in the renal pelvis is propelled by peristaltic action along the length of the ureter into the bladder. The ureters run medially and insert into the posterior base of the bladder, with the terminal end of the ureter tunnelled submucosally to form the vesicoureteric junction. The normal intrinsic musculature of the bladder surrounding the oblique course of the intravesical segment of the ureter is thought to be responsible for ureteric competence during bladder emptying, thus preventing the reflux of urine from the bladder back into the ureter. Abnormalities in the development of this intravesical segment are thought to predispose to the development of vesicoureteric reflux (see later in this chapter).

The bladder is an elastic organ consisting of connective tissue and smooth muscle, known as *detrusor*, loosely arranged in outer longitudinal, middle circular and inner longitudinal layers. This muscle arrangement results in the bladder's ability to empty during contraction. The dome of the bladder is covered by parietal peritoneum and is in apposition to other organs in the pelvis. The proximal urethra lies between the bladder neck and the pelvic diaphragm, and functionally consists of two sphincter mechanisms composed of both smooth and striated muscle. In women, the pelvic diaphragm is responsible for most of the sphincter mechanism. In men, the sphincter mechanism is largely incorporated into the prostate, with minimal sphincteric function incorporated into the bulbar and penile urethra.

Thus the kidneys and ureters are bilateral and paired, whereas the bladder and urethra are centrally placed and form a single structure. As a general principle, damage to a single kidney has minimal impact on overall renal excretory function provided the remaining kidney is normal. However, structural abnormalities of a single kidney or ureter may still predispose to infection, and may be relevant to Tommy's presentation, as will be discussed later in the chapter.

Structure of the kidney

The functional renal tissue, known as the renal parenchyma, is loosely divided into cortex and medulla. Each kidney contains about one million func-

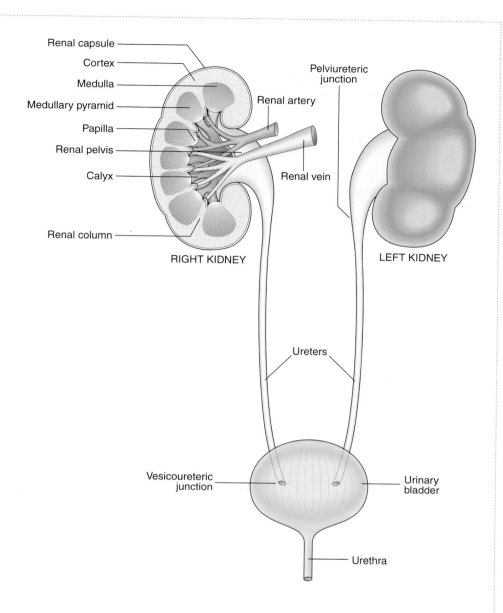

Fig. 1.1
Principal anatomical components of the urinary tract, including features seen on a cut surface of the kidney.

tional units, or nephrons, each consisting of a glomerulus and a tubule (Fig. 1.2). The glomerulus is responsible for filtering the blood, providing a barrier to the
passage of protein and red blood cells into the urine.
It is this filtrate which ultimately forms urine. After its
production in the glomerulus, the filtrate enters the
tubule, which functions to reabsorb and secrete fluid
and electrolytes to adjust the urinary composition
as necessary to maintain homeostasis of the body
fluids. All nephrons have their glomeruli located in
the cortex, which comprises the outer one-third of the
kidney. Approximately 15% of nephrons arise in the
deepest part of the cortex (the juxtamedullary area).
The inner two-thirds of the kidney consists of dark,
striated areas known as pyramids, and the intervening renal columns, which together comprise the renal
medulla. The apices of the pyramids are the renal
papillae which project into the calyces, which are
cuplike structures joining within the kidney to form
the renal pelvis.

The glomerulus consists of a network of capillaries
which invaginates the blinded end of the associated
tubule, forming the Bowman's capsule. From this
arises, in succession, the proximal tubule, the descending and ascending limbs of the loop of Henle, the
distal convoluted tubule, the cortical collecting tubule,
the outer medullary and, subsequently, the inner
medullary collecting duct, which opens at the tip of the
renal papilla into the renal pelvis. The structure and
function of the renal tubular system and glomerulus
are described in more detail in Chapters 2 and 5,
respectively.

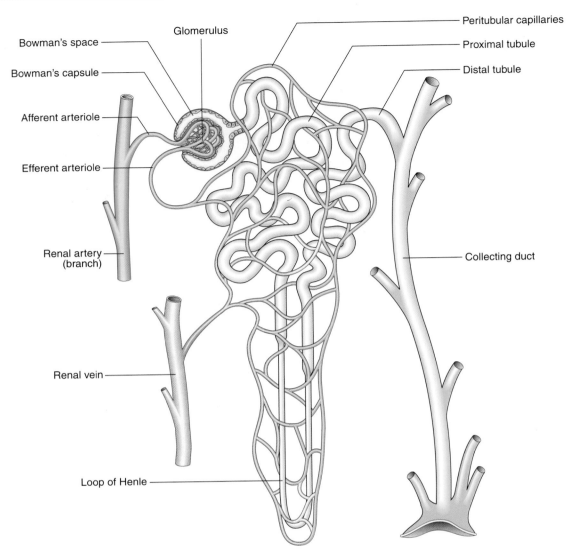

Fig. 1.2
Microscopic anatomy of the nephron showing relationship between vascular and tubular structures.

At least one renal artery supplies each kidney, but often multiple renal arteries are present. Each renal artery typically divides into five segments which subsequently branch up the sides of the pyramids, forming the interlobar arteries. At the junction of the medulla and cortex, the interlobar arteries divide into arcuate arteries. These then divide into interlobular arteries, giving rise to the afferent arterioles which feed into the glomeruli. The vessels emanating from the glomeruli are known as the efferent arterioles. The majority of efferent arterioles form a capillary network surrounding the proximal tubules within the cortex. However, the juxtamedullary glomeruli give rise to long, meshed capillary networks, the vasa recta, which participate in the countercurrent mechanism of urinary concentration in the kidney (see Chapter 3).

Innervation of the urinary tract

The neurological supply to the kidney is largely involved with regulation of vasomotor tone and hence renal blood flow. Sympathetic fibres originate in the lower splanchnic nerves and travel through the lumbar ganglion to the kidney. Stimulation of the sympathetic nervous system reduces renal blood flow by causing intrarenal vasoconstriction. It also enhances sodium reabsorption and stimulates the local renin–angiotensin system (see Chapter 2). However, denervated kidneys continue to function, usually without significant perturbations in major functional parameters.

Both sympathetic and parasympathetic nerve fibres supply the ureter. The spinal segments subtending this supply are the L1 and L2 nerve roots. Sympathetic fibres arising from the renal and intermesenteric plexuses supply the upper part of the ureter, the superior hypogastric plexus supplies the middle part, and the inferior hypogastric plexus (lying at the side of the bladder and prostate) supplies the lower part. Vagal fibres supply parasympathetic innervation to the kidney and ureter via the coeliac plexus and pelvic splanchnic nerves.

The bladder and urethra are innervated by both parasympathetic and sympathetic pathways. The parasympathetic fibres arise in the second to the fourth sacral nerve roots. They function to stimulate bladder emptying, vasodilatation and penile erection. The bladder is less densely innervated by sympathetic fibres which arise from T11–L3 nerve root segments. Stimulation of the sympathetic nervous system decreases bladder tone and inhibits the parasympathetic system. The base of the bladder and the proximal urethra are more richly innervated by sympathetic fibres which act to facilitate closure of the bladder neck and the proximal urethral sphincter. Drugs which block noradrenergic alpha-receptors (such as the antihypertensive prazosin) may inhibit periurethral sphincter function, resulting in incontinence. The pelvic diaphragm is innervated by somatic motor neurones that allow voluntary contraction and relaxation. These neurones arise from the S2–S4 segments. The pelvic diaphragm is largely responsible for maintaining continence.

The bladder distends as urine is drained into it, resulting in the maintenance of low bladder pressures. This distension is essential to prevent urinary incontinence, which will occur if bladder pressures exceed the resistance of the urethral sphincter.

Micturition is therefore a complex process of coordinated stimulation of the parasympathetic nervous system which results in bladder contraction, and inhibition of sympathetic tone which results in sphincter relaxation. Voluntary control of voiding via the somatic nervous system is essential for regular drainage of the urinary tract to occur, as well as for social and hygiene reasons.

Embryology of the kidney and urinary tract

The development *in utero* of the urinary and reproductive tracts is closely related in both males and females. In the early stages of development, the urinary and genital ducts open into a common tract or cloaca, which is the dilated portion of the hindgut (see Fig. 1.3). In men, the urinary and genital systems continue to share a common distal excretory duct system,

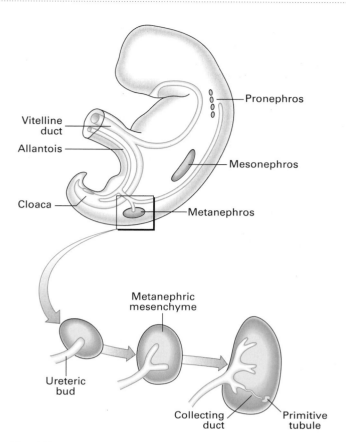

Fig. 1.3
Embryological development of the kidney.

i.e. the distal urethra. However, in women the primitive excretory duct undergoes regression and does not form part of the reproductive tract in adults.

The fetus produces and excretes urine into the allantoic or amniotic fluid sac, where it is reabsorbed. The excretory function of the kidney is not essential until after delivery. However, if developmental anomalies of the urinary tract occur, they are often detected on fetal ultrasound because of the obstructed passage of urine.

Human kidneys are derived from the sequential development of the embryonic mesodermal kidney structures: the pronephros, mesonephros and metanephros. The pronephros degenerates in embryos of about 5 mm in length before full embryonic development. The mesonephros functions for a short time *in utero* as a provisional kidney before largely degenerating into the mesonephric tubule that persists to form part of the ductal system of the male reproductive tract. The metanephros remains and develops into the functional human kidney.

The excretory part of the metanephros develops from the portion of the nephrogenic cord caudal to the mesonephros. The functional human kidney is formed by the invasion of the collecting tubules arising from the ureteric bud into the metanephric mesenchyme (Fig. 1.3). The branching and invasion of the ureteric bud into the mesenchyme is highly structured, showing several repeating patterns of division. As a result of this invasion, each tip of the branching collecting tubule has a 'cap' of approximately 100 mesenchymal cells, which are induced to survive, proliferate and undergo mesenchymal–epithelial transformation. These mesenchymal cells are effectively stem cells, capable of undergoing differentiation to form the glomeruli and the proximal, loop and distal tubular segments of the nephron. This then joins the collecting tubule derived from the ureteric bud. In addition, the metanephric mesenchyme produces non-epithelial cells that are stromal in distribution. The cells of the mesenchyme and ureteric bud also produce factors which control the growth, differentiation and migration of endothelial, mesangial, smooth muscle and interstitial cells, as well as the deposition of extra-cellular matrix. These nephrons are grouped into lobules, which persist until birth and then generally disappear. However, some lobulation may persist into adult life.

During the development of the metanephros, the kidneys undergo an upward change in position, which is due partly to the cranial growth of the ureter and partly to the diminution of body curvature. Fusion of the lower poles of the kidney during this ascent results in the defect known as horseshoe kidney.

The impact that interference with the normal development of the kidney will have on the kidney and urinary tract depends on the stage of development at which the insult occurs. During the first few weeks of embryogenesis, an injury or insult may result in congenital absence of the kidney. If the same event occurs during the second or third month of gestation, parenchymal disruption may occur. This results in cystic or hypoplastic kidneys or abnormalities of the collecting systems, such as urethral atresia, posterior urethral valves or calyceal distortion. Vestigial tubules derived from metanephric tissue which fail to join the collecting ducts may result in closed secretory loops and form renal cysts. Early separation of the ureteric bud into two or more parts may result in duplex collecting systems. Beyond the fourth month of gestation, an insult is unlikely to affect the pelvicalyceal system, as it is well defined anatomically by this stage.

The genetic and molecular basis of the processes that govern these regulated phases of renal embryonic development remain largely unknown. A number of genes, which produce a variety of molecules that may be potential regulators of renal development, have been identified. Disruption of these processes may result in a variety of developmental renal abnormalities.

One consequence of abnormal development of urinary tract structures may be impaired urinary drainage, and hence predisposition to infection. This possibility will be explored in relation to our febrile child.

Urinary tract structure and infection box 2

Tommy's test results

Tommy's blood tests demonstrated a high white cell count of 23.0×10^9/L* with a neutrophilia (increased neutrophil count) of 85%, suggestive of bacterial sepsis. The overall filtration function of his kidneys was normal, reflected by a serum creatinine concentration of 45 μmol/L. Blood and urine cultures were taken, and he was started on intravenous fluids and antibiotics. His urine culture subsequently demonstrated a pure growth of *E. coli*.

This information confirms the suspicion that Tommy has a urinary infection. We now need to consider the following issues.

① Is it normal for microorganisms to be present in the urinary tract?

② What are the factors that protect against organisms entering and infecting the urinary tract?

③ How is urinary tract infection diagnosed?

(*Values are outside the normal range; see Appendix.)

Infection of the urinary tract

Infection of the urinary tract is one of the most common bacterial infections in both children and adults. The clinical features, diagnosis, treatment and significance of the infection vary depending on the site of infection and the presence or absence of structural and/or functional abnormalities within the urinary tract. Recurrent urinary infection, when complicated by major structural abnormalities, can lead to chronic renal failure. In the presence of underlying kidney disease, superimposed infection often accelerates functional decline. However, recurrent uncomplicated urinary infection, although common and debilitating, generally has no long-term deleterious consequences.

Asymptomatic bacteriuria

Asymptomatic bacteriuria is defined as the presence of bacteria in the urinary tract in the absence of symptoms attributable to infection. Contamination of urine by organisms normally residing in the female periurethral area at the time of collection is common. Thus it is generally considered that 'significant bacteriuria' is present when 10^5 or more of the same organisms per millilitre are present in two voided urinary specimens (or in one 'in–out' catheter specimen) in a woman, or in one voided specimen in a man. In general, antibiotic treatment of asymptomatic bacteriuria is only indicated in the presence of factors leading to potentially complicated urinary infection (including pregnancy). In many circumstances, asymptomatic bacteriuria is a recurrent problem and antibiotic therapy may lead to antibiotic resistance that may cause infection to be more difficult to eradicate.

Acute urinary tract infection

Acute infection of the urinary tract can generally be divided on clinical grounds into upper or lower tract infection (Table 1.1).

The clinical presentation of urinary tract infection in children is much more variable and is frequently non-specific, as in Tommy's case. Thus children may present with lethargy, vomiting, fever, poor weight gain, irritability, febrile convulsions or gastrointestinal symptoms. Hence, the diagnosis should be considered in any sick infant or toddler.

Another basis of classification is whether the infection is 'complicated' (by systemic or anatomical abnormalities; Table 1.2) or 'uncomplicated'.

Lower urinary tract infections are particularly common in women, where they are generally localized to the bladder (cystitis). In adult men, the urethra and/or the prostate may be the primary site of infection. In the latter instances, sexually transmitted disease should be considered, particularly if no overt infection is isolated on urine culture (see below).

Upper urinary tract infection is defined as infection involving the kidney. As the renal pelvis is invariably involved in ascending infection, this is also referred to as acute pyelonephritis.

These arbitrary divisions have implications for treatment and prognosis, and guide decisions regarding further investigation. If the kidneys and urinary tract are normal anatomically and functionally, infection is unlikely to result in significant renal impairment, even when persistent and/or recurrent. However, if there is impaired renal function, reduced systemic resistance to infection, or abnormal drainage of the urinary tract, an infection is likely to become complicated, with the risk of renal damage, abscess formation or septicaemia. As dilatation and impaired drainage of the urinary tract is inevitable in pregnancy, all urinary infection in pregnant women should be treated as a potentially complicated infection.

Aetiology and pathogenesis of urinary tract infection

There are numerous differences in the clinical features, response to therapy and prognosis of urinary infection according to the age of the patient, site of infection and whether the infection is complicated or uncomplicated. However, the microbial aetiology of infections is similar throughout the urinary system regardless of clinical setting.

Bacteria are by far the most common cause of urinary infection, with most other infecting organisms occurring in patients with underlying systemic illness (Table 1.3).

E. coli accounts for approximately 85% of community-acquired and 50% of hospital-acquired urinary infection. However, almost every organism has been associated with urinary tract infection, especially in

Table 1.1
Clinical features of acute lower and upper urinary tract infection in adults

Lower urinary tract infection	Upper urinary tract infection*
Dysuria	Systemically unwell
Frequency	Fever ± rigors
Suprapubic pain	Loin pain and tenderness
Malodorous urine	Nausea and vomiting
Haematuria	Hypotension or shock
Normal temperature	±Features of lower urinary tract infection

*Acute infection of the upper urinary tract is also referred to as acute pyelonephritis.

Table 1.2
Underlying factors associated with 'complicated' urinary tract infection

Systemic conditions
 Diabetes mellitus
 Papillary necrosis (e.g. analgesic nephropathy)
 Immunodeficient states (including immunosuppressive drug therapy)
Abnormal drainage of urine
 Renal calculi
 Urinary obstruction
 Vesicoureteric reflux
 Pelviureteric junction obstruction
 Instrumentation of the urinary tract (including catheters)
 Pregnancy

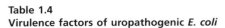
Table 1.3
Microbiological agents causing urinary tract infection

Community-acquired	Hospital-acquired
Escherichia coli	Escherichia coli
Klebsiella spp.	Klebsiella spp.
Proteus mirabilis	Citrobacter spp.
Staphylococcus saprophyticus	Enterobacter spp.
	Pseudomonas aeruginosa
	Enterococcus faecalis
	Coagulase-negative Staphylococcus spp.
	Candida spp.*

*These are yeasts (fungi).

Table 1.4
Virulence factors of uropathogenic *E. coli*

Lower urinary tract
 Rapid growth rate
 Adhesion to uroepithelial cells (bacterial fimbriae)
 Endotoxin production (lipopolysaccharide)
Upper urinary tract
 Resistance to serum bactericidal activity
 Siderophore and haemolysin production
 Resistance to phagocytosis
 Persistence of organism within the kidney

the immunocompromised inpatient population and in those with urological instrumentation. Organisms not traditionally regarded as urological pathogens may also occur in this population in whom natural host defence mechanisms are compromised. These organisms include lactobacilli, *Gardnerella vaginalis* and mycoplasma species, including *Ureaplasma urealyticum*. Staphylococcal pyelonephritis (almost always *S. aureus*) should always raise the possibility of haematogenous spread from distant foci as this is an unusual organism to colonize the periurethra and cause ascending infection.

Most episodes of urinary sepsis are caused by ascending infection, with a small percentage of upper urinary infections arising from the haematogenous (bloodborne) route. The vaginal introitus is normally colonized with a variety of non-virulent streptococci, staphylococci and lactobacilli, which are only occasionally responsible for urinary infection. Gram-negative bacteria, which are much more likely to cause urinary infection, normally reside in the bowel and colonize the introitus in a proportion of women. Factors thought to be responsible for periurethral colonization by colonic bacteria and subsequent bacterial entry into the bladder include previous antibiotic therapy, the use of a diaphragm and spermicide for contraceptive purposes, and sexual activity. In many instances an alteration in sexual activity (either sexual partner or frequency of intercourse) will predispose to urinary infection in women.

Different factors operate to prevent urinary infection at each anatomical level in the urinary tract. The common uropathogens are able to overcome the normal host defence mechanisms that protect against urinary infection. The relative contribution of bacterial virulence factors to infection depends on the site of infection as well as the normality or otherwise of the urinary tract. In the presence of an anatomically abnormal urinary tract, organisms of low

virulence may still be able to establish a significant infection. However, this is rarely the case if such organisms infect a structurally normal urinary tract. Under normal circumstances bacteria introduced into the bladder are rapidly cleared by the constant urine flow, which serves to flush the bladder and dilute its contents. The direct antibacterial properties of the urine and of the bladder mucosa, as well as urinary constituents (such as high osmolarity, urea and organic acids), inhibit bacterial growth in the urine. However, the presence of glucose and amino acids may facilitate bacterial growth. Prostatic secretions have bactericidal properties, and white cells within the bladder mucosa participate in local defence against infection.

Bacterial virulence factors have been best studied in *E. coli* (Table 1.4), where a limited number of serotypes have been found to be responsible for the majority of infections. Various antigenic factors have been identified which enhance the urovirulence of a particular strain.

The adherence of *E. coli* to urothelial cells is predominantly determined by bacterial fimbriae, which are filamentous processes projecting from the cell surface. In addition, the capsules of *E. coli* contain specific virulence factors. Capsular antigens possess antiphagocytic activity and are important when tissue invasion occurs. As iron is a necessary bacterial nutrient, mechanisms to chelate and scavenge iron efficiently (siderophores) confer increased pathogenicity. Similarly, bacterial haemolysin production, which facilitates the release of haem, increases iron scavenging and thus virulence.

Urease production by organisms such as *Proteus mirabilis*, *P. vulgaris* and *S. saprophyticus* is involved in tissue adherence, and also in splitting urea into carbon dioxide and ammonia. This urease activity results in urinary alkalinization and precipitation of magnesium, ammonium and phosphate. Thus infection with these organisms often becomes complicated by stone formation (struvite).

Investigation of urinary tract infection

The laboratory diagnosis of urinary tract infection depends on microbiological confirmation of infection. This is usually taken to mean a bacterial count of greater than 10^5 colony-forming units (CFU) per millilitre. The technique of collection of the urine specimen is critical. In men the collection of a midstream specimen is usually successful and contamination is rare. In women, the introitus should be cleaned with saline (not antiseptic as this may inhibit bacterial growth and cause a falsely negative culture result). A midstream urine is collected with the labia spread apart. Collection in infants and children is difficult as adhesive bags are likely to become contaminated. In these circumstances suprapubic aspiration is a safe alternative that provides a definitive diagnosis. Urine can be stored at 4°C for up to 48h before culture.

Although the laboratory cut-off for significant infection is regarded as 10^5 CFU/mL, infection may be present when colony counts are between 10^2 and 10^5 CFU/mL, particularly in the case of less common organisms such as Gram-positive bacteria and some fungi. Mixed cultures, particularly in the presence of low colony counts in females, are usually the result of contamination.

Because of the delay inherent in microbiological confirmation of urinary tract infection, urinalysis is often used as a first line screen in individuals with symptoms suggestive of urinary infection (Fig. 1.4).

Biochemical reagent strips will detect nitrites, which are produced by common uropathogens, and also leucocytes. The finding of pyuria (increased leucocyte excretion) does not always correlate with infection, since it may occur with other causes of urogenital inflammation and in normal pregnancy. Microscopic haematuria and proteinuria on urinalysis may be indicative of urinary tract inflammation, but are unreliable as markers of infection when additional renal or urinary tract pathology is present. Urine microscopy may demonstrate red cells, white cells and bacteria characteristic of infection. Evidence of white cell casts is suggestive of renal parenchymal infection. Additional tests have been developed to localize the site of infection to the upper or lower urinary tract, but these are not routinely used in clinical practice. In patients presenting with systemic features of pyelonephritis, septicaemia is possible and, in this clinical setting, blood should be taken for culture.

In otherwise healthy sexually active women, isolated lower urinary infection in the absence of systemic or structural factors predisposing to complicated infection (see Table 1.2) requires no further investigation. Urinary infection in males should be regarded as being potentially complicated, and underlying abnormalities of the urinary tract, particularly those causing obstruction of urine flow, should be sought. In younger males, congenital abnormalities of the urinary tract predominate, including vesicoureteric reflux and the presence of urethral valves, while in older males, bladder neck

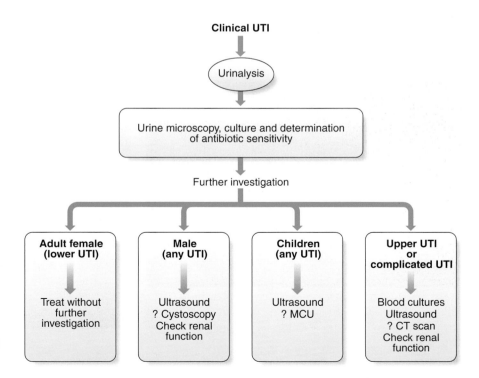

Fig. 1.4
Patterns of investigation in urinary tract infection. MCU, micturating cystourethrogram; UTI, urinary tract infection.

9

obstruction caused by prostatic hypertrophy or ure-thral stricture is more likely. Further imaging investigations are necessary in these cases, as in any patient with complicated or upper urinary tract infection.

> ### Urinary tract structure and infection box 3
>
> **The next step**
>
> The severity of the systemic features in Tommy's case suggest that an underlying abnormality of the urinary tract may account for the infection. Indeed, the above discussion would suggest that, if free drainage of the urinary tract existed, infection is unlikely to have taken hold, particularly in a male.
>
> In light of Tommy's age, the most likely underlying cause is a congenital abnormality of the urinary tract. In an older person, acquired abnormalities of the urinary tract are more commonly found. The nature of the structural abnormality is often easily determined by simple imaging of the urinary tract. This raises the issue of what techniques are available to gain a view of the anatomy of the urinary tract in different clinical settings.

Imaging of the urinary tract

Renal ultrasound is the initial screening test used for imaging the urinary tract in children, in men or in the presence of complicated infection. It will define whether urinary tract dilatation is present and whether the underlying renal size and parenchymal thickness is normal (Fig. 1.5). The level of obstruction is suggested but the result may not be definitive, and intravenous pyelography (IVP) may be indicated subsequently (Fig. 1.6). If abscess formation is suspected, computed tomography (CT scanning) may be required to define the intrarenal mass as well as to monitor the response to therapy.

IVP is rarely, if ever, indicated in the acute setting and, with the increasing expertise in ultrasonography, it is only occasionally performed as a follow-up investigation. Its main value is to provide a functional and anatomical assessment of drainage of the urinary tract, particularly after correction of obstructive pathology.

A radionuclide blood flow scan is of use in assessing renal perfusion (see Chapter 9) and avoids exposure to potentially nephrotoxic contrast agents.

Cystoscopy (direct inspection of the interior of the bladder) should be performed if primary bladder or prostate pathology is suspected. It is rarely indicated in patients with urinary infection who have normal upper tracts demonstrated on ultrasound. If impaired bladder function is suspected, urodynamic studies which record changes in pressure during bladder filling and emptying may be indicated.

All children presenting with urinary infection should be investigated with imaging of the urinary tract since up to 50% will be found to have a urological abnormality. In the majority of these children, vesicoureteric reflux (see below) will be confirmed. In infants who are acutely unwell with pyelonephritis, both ultrasound and micturating cystourethrogram (MCU) should be performed. The MCU demonstrates the presence of backflow of urine from the bladder into the ureters during micturition (vesicoureteric reflux).

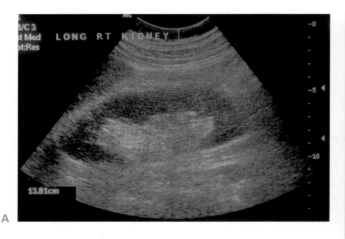

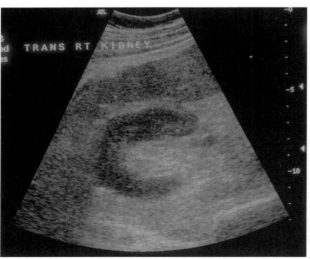

Fig. 1.5

Normal renal ultrasound (long axis (A) and transverse axis (B) views).

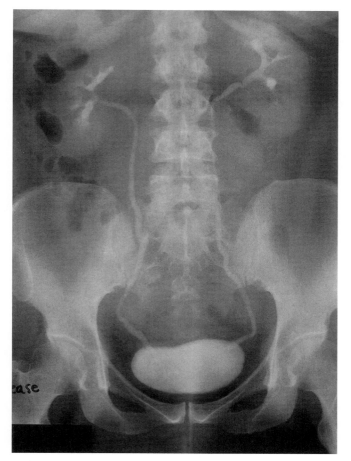

Fig. 1.6
Normal intravenous pyelogram.

Diagnosis and management

Soon after admission, Tommy underwent renal ultrasonography, which showed that the right kidney was 2 cm smaller than the left, with generalized loss of cortical thickness. The pelvis and ureter were dilated down to the level of the vesicoureteric junction but no obstruction was demonstrated. The right ureteric insertion into the bladder was laterally placed, and ureteric 'jets' (indicating normal pulsatile flow of urine from the ureter to the bladder) were not seen. This was taken as evidence of an abnormality of the vesicoureteric junction on that side. No abnormality was observed in the left kidney, pelvis or collecting system, and a normal left ureteric insertion and ureteric jets were noted.

After starting antibiotics (ceftriaxone), Tommy became afebrile with improved appetite over the ensuing 72 h. Intravenous antibiotics were continued for a total of 7 days, after which he was given oral cefaclor for a further week. Tommy was subsequently maintained on a preventative dose of trimethoprim/sulfamethoxazole at night. A repeat urine culture 3 weeks after his initial presentation was sterile.

It was recommended that his two siblings, aged 5 and 7 years, who were asymptomatic, should undergo screening urine culture and ultrasonography for the detection of vesicoureteric reflux.

It is clear that an underlying anatomical abnormality has contributed to Tommy's infection. Vesicoureteric reflux is one of the commonest congenital abnormalities of the urogenital tract. The following questions are likely to be raised by Tommy's parents and will be discussed:

① What causes vesicoureteric reflux?

② How is it diagnosed?

③ What treatment is indicated?

In older children an MCU is not always considered necessary in the presence of a good quality ultrasound view of the upper urinary tract, with visualization of the ureteric orifices and ureteric peristalsis. A radionuclide scan using DMSA (dimercaptosuccinic acid) is performed to detect renal parenchymal scarring (Fig. 1.7). This is not generally undertaken within 6–12 months of acute pyelonephritis to avoid false positive results.

See box 4.

Vesicoureteric reflux

Vesicoureteric reflux (VUR) is caused by incompetence of the vesicoureteric junction. In most instances the defect is one of shortness of the submucosal segment because of lateral ectopia (displacement) of the ureteric orifice. This results in loss of the normal valvelike action associated with the oblique path of the terminal segment of ureter through the bladder wall (Fig. 1.8).

In the majority of infants, VUR presents with a complicating urinary infection. However, signs localizing the infection to the urinary tract may not always be present, especially in the very young. In males particularly, infection may not always occur, and more subtle signs of renal damage caused by retrograde urine flow (reflux nephropathy) may be present (Table 1.5).

If enuresis (bed-wetting) persists until after primary school age (10 years), reflux should be excluded with renal ultrasonography. Enuresis in this setting is caused by the presence of residual urine after

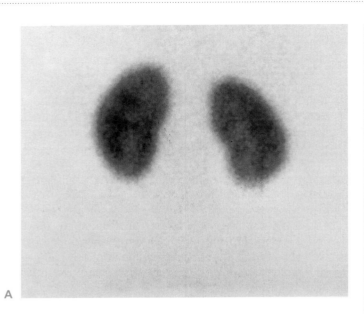

A

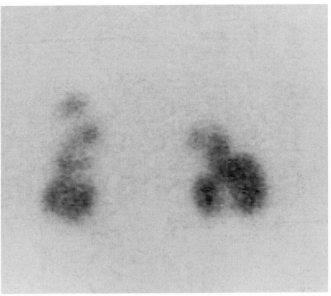

B

Fig. 1.7

(A) Normal dimercaptosuccinic acid (DMSA) renal scan; (B) DMSA renal scan showing multiple cortical defects and severe bilateral renal scarring, worse in the upper pole.

Table 1.5
Features of vesicoureteric reflux and reflux nephropathy

Vesicoureteric reflux	Reflux nephropathy
Ultrasound *in utero* (incidental finding)	Hypertension
	Proteinuria
Enuresis	Renal impairment
Double voiding	Impaired urine concentration
Loin pain on micturition	*with or without features of VUR*
Urinary tract infection	
Family screening	

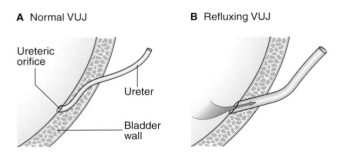

A Normal VUJ

B Refluxing VUJ

Ureteric orifice

Ureter

Bladder wall

Fig. 1.8

Vesicoureteric junction (VUJ): (**A**) normal; (**B**) defective, with reflux.

voiding as the upper urinary tract empties into the bladder, and also by impaired tubular function with loss of the ability to concentrate the urine which leads to increased urine volumes. In adults, enuresis rarely persists but nocturia may be a prominent symptom.

It has recently been recognized that reflux nephropathy is inherited as an autosomal dominant condition. Thus current recommendations advise routine ultrasound in neonates of parents known to have reflux nephropathy independent of the grade of reflux in the affected parent.

The diagnosis of VUR is based on demonstration of reflux on an MCU or real time ultrasound. There may also be radiological findings of focal scarring in the kidneys, generally at the upper pole, with calyceal clubbing. If more severe VUR is present, the kidney may be diffusely damaged with generalized loss of parenchymal tissue (Fig. 1.9).

VUR is the commonest underlying cause of hypertension in children and is associated with the presence of renal scarring. VUR may present in adults with moderate to severe hypertension without a history of urinary infection. Renal calculi are commonly present in areas of scarring within the kidney and presumably relate to urinary stasis. Urinary infection with *P. mirabilis* or other urea-splitting organisms may be associated with staghorn calculi but, with appropriate early treatment of infection with antibiotics, this is a relatively rare complication.

Antireflux surgery to correct the incompetence of the vesicoureteric junction is not generally recommended unless severe reflux causing upper tract dilatation is present. Corrective surgery is not undertaken after 2–3 years of age. It has long been appreciated that once renal parenchymal scarring is present, even in unilateral reflux, antireflux surgery does not protect against progressive decline in renal function.

Overall, reflux nephropathy accounts for approximately 8% of patients with end-stage renal failure in Australia and New Zealand, and 20–25% of the paediatric population with end-stage renal failure. Reflux nephropathy with progressive functional deterioration is characterized by hypertension and persistent proteinuria, which is a poor prognostic feature.

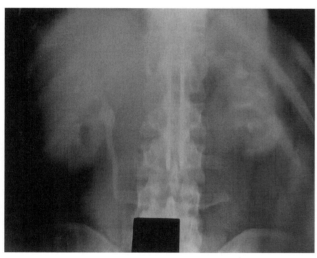

Fig. 1.9
Intravenous pyelogram showing gross scarring of left kidney, with clubbing of calyces characteristic of reflux nephropathy. Normal right kidney and collecting system.

Follow-up

At review 12 months later, Tommy's urine remains sterile with no proteinuria, and his growth and milestones appear normal. His blood pressure is at the upper limit of normal at 90/60 mmHg. Repeat renal ultrasound is unchanged from that performed during the acute phase of his illness, although the right renal parenchyma is now less oedematous and the kidney measures 2.5 cm smaller than the left. A DMSA scan is performed which shows diffuse parenchymal cortical scars on the right, but none in the left kidney.

The management plan for Tommy is to maintain the prophylactic antibiotic until he is 5 years of age, and then repeat the ultrasound and DMSA scan. In the absence of new scar formation, it is planned that antibiotics will be ceased at that stage. Regular follow-up of blood pressure and urinalyses are advised to detect any increase in urinary protein excretion.

His 7-year-old sister has sterile urine, but renal ultrasonography and subsequent DMSA scan are suggestive of a right upper pole scar. There is no ultrasound evidence of ongoing reflux, with ureteric peristalsis and ureteric jets appearing normal. The management plan is to have 6-monthly urinalyses and a repeat DMSA scan in 1 year. In the absence of infection and progressive renal scarring, her blood pressure and urinalysis will be monitored on a 2–3-yearly basis. The risks of infection in pregnancy and potential for developing hypertension, particularly in pregnancy, are explained to her mother for future information. The remaining sibling is normal.

Overview: treatment of urinary tract infections

Most episodes of uncomplicated lower urinary tract infection are isolated events affecting sexually active women. Suitable antibiotics for use in this setting include trimethoprim, cefalexin and amoxicillin/ clavulanate. In most cases, a 3-day course of therapy provides adequate treatment. In relapsing infection, a 10–14-day course of antibiotics should be prescribed and if infection persists or recurs investigation should be undertaken. Recurrent infection (more than three episodes per year) is best treated with prophylactic low-dose antibiotics. However, in patients with a clear relation between infection and sexual activity, single dose therapy after intercourse may be effective. Generally, follow-up cultures are not needed in otherwise uncomplicated urinary infection.

The treatment of acute upper urinary tract infection (acute pyelonephritis) is generally performed in hospital. Intravenous fluids and empiric antibiotic treatment (e.g. intravenous cephalothin) should be commenced before culture results become available.

An appropriate oral antibiotic may be substituted when the fever subsides. The total duration of antibiotic treatment is generally 2 weeks. If no significant improvement is observed within 48 h, the diagnosis and choice of antibiotic therapy should be reviewed, and imaging of the kidney undertaken to exclude obstruction or abscess.

Self-assessment case study

A 24-year-old woman presents at 28 weeks' gestation with frequency and dysuria. On examination she looks relatively well. She is afebrile, but her blood pressure is elevated at 145/95 mmHg. She has mild suprapubic tenderness but no loin tenderness. Urinalysis and subsequent culture are consistent with urinary tract infection and cephalosporin treatment is prescribed.

Upon review of her antenatal history, asymptomatic bacteriuria had been detected at her booking-in visit at 8 weeks' gestation. This was treated with a 7-day course of antibiotics. A follow-up urine culture was not performed. Her blood pressure had been 140/95 at both 8 and 12 weeks' gestation and 140/90 at 18 weeks. At a visit at 12 weeks' gestation no urinary infection was detected and urinalysis demonstrated proteinuria +.

Her past history included an episode of kidney infection at age 11 years, at which time a horseshoe kidney was diagnosed. She was told that her kidney functioned normally and no specific follow-up was recommended. She had enuresis till the age of 12 years, as did her sister, and has had nocturia on a regular basis for as long as she can recall.

After studying this chapter you should be able to answer the following questions.

① What are the key clinical features suggestive of underlying urinary tract abnormality in this case?

② What tests would have been done to confirm infection in this young woman?

③ Is it likely that she currently has a lower or upper urinary tract infection? What factors predispose her to developing a complicated (or upper urinary tract) infection?

④ What recommendations would you make about her current treatment and what follow-up investigations would you perform after the delivery of her child?

Answers see page 144

Self-assessment questions

① Can you describe the major anatomical components of the urinary tract?

② Describe the embryological derivation of the major structures of the kidney.

③ Describe the mechanisms that normally protect the urinary tract from infection.

④ What are the principles of treatment of (i) uncomplicated lower urinary tract infection and (ii) upper urinary tract infection?

Answers see page 144

BODY FLUIDS AND NEPHRON FUNCTION

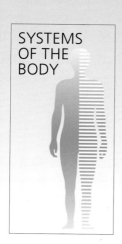

SYSTEMS
OF THE
BODY

Chapter objectives

After studying this chapter you should be able to:

① Describe the normal distribution and composition of body fluids.

② Give some causes and clinical features of hypovolaemia and hypervolaemia.

③ Describe the functional anatomy of the nephron.

④ Give an account of the main sodium transport processes in the nephron, and the normal regulation of sodium and potassium excretion.

⑤ Describe the site and mechanism of action of commonly used diuretic drugs.

⑥ Outline some common disturbances of sodium and potassium balance.

Introduction

The main function of the kidney is not 'to produce urine' (this is an inconvenience rather than a biological necessity), but to regulate the volume and composition of the body fluids within narrow limits. While the best known task performed by the kidney is filtration of the blood, this is really just the first step in a sequence of actions whereby the functional unit of the kidney, the nephron, responds to disturbances in the volume and composition of the circulating fluids. This results in the excretion of urine as a byproduct.

While many types of kidney disease can interfere with these processes, significant alterations in nephron function can be produced even in a person with normal kidneys by pharmacological agents which interfere with the normal physiological mechanisms operating in the nephron. As illustrated by the case discussed in this chapter, this can have serious impli-cations for the volume and electrolyte composition of the plasma.

See box 1.

Body fluid and electrolyte distribution

A number of features of Joanne's history and physical examination suggest that her total body fluid volume is reduced. First, her symptoms of light-headedness and near-fainting attacks suggest that her cardiovascular system is unable to maintain perfusion of her brain, especially when she is upright. This inference is confirmed on physical examination, where it is found that she has a lowish lying blood pressure which falls further on standing, accompanied by a marked increase in her pulse rate. These features are suggestive of activated sympathetic nervous system responses to maintain her cardiac output in the face of

---

Body fluids and nephron function box 1

Fluid and electrolyte depletion

Joanne Smithfield is a 19-year-old woman who presents to her family doctor complaining of weakness and light-headedness. These symptoms have been troubling her for some 6 months, but in the last week she has become more concerned as she has had a number of near-fainting episodes at work. These attacks are usually initiated by getting up rapidly from her desk, which makes her feel light-headed until she sits or lies down again. She has also noticed increasing difficulty walking up the stairs in her block of flats, where she lives with a girlfriend on the second floor. She attrib-utes this to weakness in her legs, though she had pre-viously been a strong runner at school.

Joanne's past medical history is unremarkable. Her menarche (commencement of menstruation) was at age 11 years, and her periods have been regular in timing and moderate in volume. She mentioned that she had gained too much weight as an adolescent, but considered that this was now 'under control'. Her family history includes hypertension and heart failure diagnosed recently in her father, but her mother is well at age 48 years and is a fitness instructor. She has a younger sister who is a keen athlete. Joanne smokes 10 cigarettes/day and drinks a little alcohol after work on some days and on weekends. Her only medications are occasional laxatives when she gets constipated, and 'fluid tablets' to remove puffiness around her ankles which she thinks makes her look unattractive.

On physical examination, Joanne looks well though a little tired. She takes a few moments to stand up from her chair, and steadies herself against the wall after doing so. Her tongue and mouth appear rather dry, and her skin feels quite doughy. Her blood pressure is 105/70 lying, 95/70 sitting, 85/65 standing. The pulse rate increases from 85 beats/min lying to 105 beats/min standing. Heart sounds are normal, and the lung fields are clear. Abdominal examination is unremarkable, although some stretch marks are noted. Neurological examination reveals normal cranial nerves, but moder-ate weakness proximally in the upper and lower limbs. Reflexes and sensory testing are normal.

At the end of the examination, Joanne is questioned further about her use of diuretic tablets. She confesses that lately she has been taking one or two furosemide (frusemide; Lasix) tablets daily, as she finds this helps to keep her weight down and avoid swelling around her ankles and hips. She initially obtained these from her father, but subsequently got them from a friend who is prescribed them by her family doctor for premen-strual swelling.

In response to this presentation we can ask the questions:

① What physiological disturbances are causing Joanne's symptoms?

② How might these disturbances have come about?

a low circulating fluid volume. Her dry mouth and flaccid skin are suggestive of depletion of mucosal and tissue water, consistent with dehydration.

A summary of clinical features of hypovolaemia (sometimes loosely called dehydration, which strictly refers to a pure water deficit) contrasted with features typically found in hypervolaemia (also called fluid overload) is given in Table 2.1. As will be explained further below, these disturbances come about more through underlying disturbances of body sodium content than from primary changes in body water.

Since we suspect that something has depleted Joanne's body of fluid, we need to ask this question: how is water normally distributed within the body, and what is the composition of the fluid in different body compartments?

Body fluid compartments

The total body water content for a typical adult is approximately 60% of the lean body mass, i.e. about 40 litres in an average 70 kg man. This can be determined by studying the dilution of marker substances which are known to distribute into all compartments of the body water.

The most familiar fraction of body fluid, namely the blood, represents a relatively small compartment of the total body water. Indeed, Fig. 2.1 shows that some 62.5% (5/8ths) of the total body water is actually located inside cells (the intracellular fluid or ICF), while 37.5% (3/8ths) is in the extracellular fluid compartment (ECF). Furthermore, the plasma component of the blood accounts for a relatively small part (around 20%) of the ECF, with the remainder being distributed as interstitial fluid (ISF) within the various organs and tissues of the body but outside the cells. It can also be seen from Fig. 2.1 that the blood is actually

composed in part of ECF (the plasma component) and in part ICF (the red cells).

In a normal individual, the volumes in the various body fluid compartments are remarkably constant in the face of somewhat variable water intake from one day to another. This constancy, an example of the *homeostasis* of the body's internal environment, is dependent on a number of finely tuned regulatory mechanisms which will be outlined in this and the next chapter, and in other books in this series. In brief, a state of equilibrium (or balance) is achieved such that the net intake of water, largely by mouth under normal circumstances, is matched by the total losses through the skin, lungs, gut and kidneys. Typical volumes involved in these fluxes on a daily basis are shown in Fig. 2.2. It is important to understand that the major control mechanism for adjusting water loss from the body to match daily water intake resides in the kidney. The kidney has a highly regulated capacity to vary the daily output of urine, while losses from the other sites are largely fixed.

Body fluid composition

There are important differences in the solute composition of the various compartments of body fluid, and these have major implications for normal cell metabolism, and for the normal function of the circulatory and neuromuscular systems.

The major features of the chemical make-up of the ICF and the ECF (the latter having two major subdivisions, the plasma and the interstitial fluid) are shown in Fig. 2.3.

Table 2.1
Clinical features of hypovolaemia and hypervolaemia

	Hypovolaemia	*Hypervolaemia*
Symptoms	Thirst	Ankle swelling
	Dizziness on standing	Breathlessness
	Confusion	
Signs	Low JVP	Oedema
	Postural hypotension	Raised JVP
	Dry mouth	Pulmonary crepitations
	Reduced skin turgor	Hypertension (sometimes)
	Reduced urine output	Weight gain
	Weight loss	

JVP, jugular venous pressure.

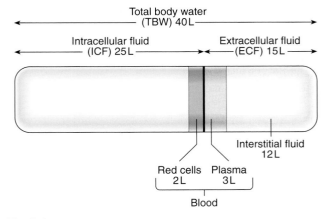

Fig. 2.1
Compartments of distribution of total body water. Approximate volumes (in litres) are shown for an average adult.

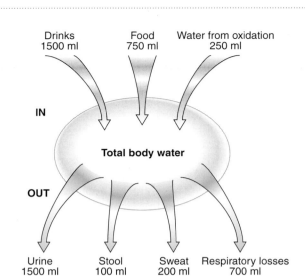

Fig. 2.2
Typical fluxes involved in daily water balance.

In brief, the main distinction between the ICF and the ECF is that the dominant cation in the ECF is sodium (Na^+) while in the ICF it is potassium (K^+). Chloride and bicarbonate make up most of the balancing anions in the ECF, while in the ICF the principal negative charges are carried by phosphate and other organic anions. In addition, there is an important contribution to the intracellular anion pool from negative charges on the many cellular proteins contained in that compartment. There is normally a zero net flux of water across the cell membrane, i.e. the ECF and ICF are in 'osmotic equilibrium'.

The mechanism for establishing and maintaining this substantial gradient for cations between the interior and exterior of cells is the membrane-bound sodium–potassium 'pump' (Na,K-activated ATPase). This ubiquitous active transport carrier uses energy derived directly from the hydrolysis of ATP to extrude three sodium ions from the cell for every two potassium ions it takes up from the ECF. The pump itself thus contributes towards generating the inside-

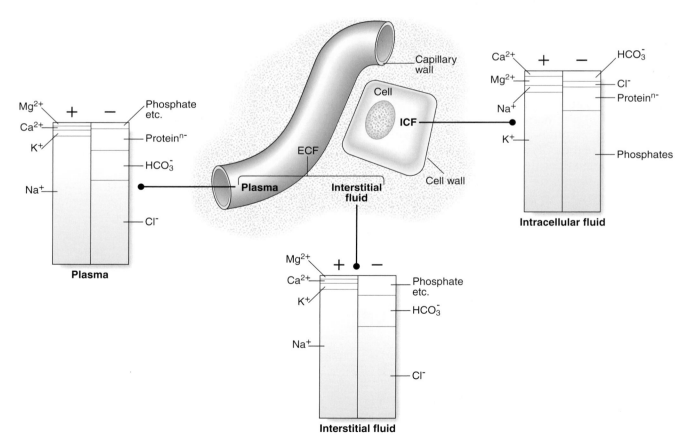

Fig. 2.3
Chemical composition of different compartments of body water. ICF, intracellular fluid; ECF, extracellular fluid.

negative membrane potential of the cell. A further contribution comes from the back-diffusion of intracellular potassium ions to the cell exterior through potassium channels present in the cell membrane.

The significance of the gradient for Na and K maintained across cell membranes in all body tissues is profound. First, high intracellular K concentrations are essential for the normal operation of many enzyme systems which drive cell metabolism. Second, the basis of electrical excitability of neuromuscular and cardiac membranes is the presence of steep concentration gradients for Na and K across these membranes. Third, the capacity of epithelia which line interfaces between the body and the exterior to carry out net transepithelial solute transport depends on the maintenance of Na and K gradients in cells of these tissues. In the last case, however, the pump units are asymmetrically distributed in opposing cell membrane surfaces (illustrated for the kidney later in this chapter).

Another important distinction is that existing between the composition of the plasma and ISF components of the ECF. As shown in Fig. 2.3, the main difference here is that the plasma, but not the ISF, contains a substantial concentration of proteins, comprising both serum albumin as well as a spectrum of globulins.

The mechanism for maintaining this protein differential within the subsections of the ECF is the presence of a permeability barrier at the capillary wall which largely prevents the movement of proteins out of the capillaries under normal circumstances.

The significance of this protein concentration gradient is that it makes an important contribution to the balance of forces across the capillary wall (specifically to the colloid osmotic – or oncotic – pressure of the plasma), favouring fluid retention within the capillaries, thus maintaining an adequate circulating plasma volume. The effect of disturbance of this gradient will be illustrated in the discussion of oedema states in Chapter 6 of this volume.

The central importance of sodium for stability of the circulation

From the above discussion it is clear that sodium is the dominant ionic species in the ECF since, together with its accompanying anions, it accounts for over 95% of the solute present in this fluid compartment. This is equivalent to saying that sodium is responsible for nearly all of the osmotic activity in the ECF (the 'oncotic' pressure attributable to plasma proteins, referred to above, is much smaller, though it is important as a differential osmotic force across capillary

membranes). Thus, when water is added to the body, the amount held in the ECF is largely determined by the body's sodium content, since the great majority of sodium ions are confined to the ECF compartment.

This gives rise to the important clinical deduction that factors which deplete the body of sodium will be associated with a low ECF volume (and hence of circulating plasma), while sodium retention is associated with expanded ECF volume. A summary of the causes of hypovolaemia and hypervolaemia based on sodium disturbances is given in Table 2.2. Note that pure disturbances in body mechanisms for regulating water itself are relatively uncommon causes of these conditions, but are more likely to produce changes in plasma sodium concentration and osmolality (see Chapter 3).

Body fluids and nephron function box 2

A probable culprit

So far we can deduce from the cardiovascular clues in the history and physical examination that Joanne has probably experienced a reduction in the circulating component of the ECF, namely the plasma. The dryness of her mouth and laxity of her skin suggest that other tissue fluid compartments are also depleted of water.

While a number of causes for this situation may be considered, in this case we have the information that she has been taking a drug which is intended to cause the kidneys to excrete higher than normal volumes of urine, causing her total body water content to be reduced.

A number of new questions now arise related to the role of the kidney in the origin of Joanne's problem, namely:

① How does the kidney normally make urine?

② How has the diuretic drug interfered with these processes to lead to body fluid depletion?

Functional anatomy of the nephron

In fundamental terms, the kidney provides a site of interface between the circulating blood and the outside world. At this interface, a number of regulatory processes occur which allow for a finely tuned response by the kidney to signals concerning the volume and composition of the circulating plasma, leading to the excretion from the body of urine whose volume and composition represent a byproduct of these processes.

The functional unit in which these interchanges are carried out within the kidney is the nephron. It is a microscopic structure consisting of a glomerulus, or 'small ball' of capillaries derived from the renal arterial supply, closely associated with an elongated tube-like structure (the tubular system) which is lined by a single layer of epithelial cells.

As shown schematically in Fig. 2.4, the two fundamental steps in nephron function are glomerular filtration, and modification of the filtered fluid as it passes through the tubular system.

Table 2.2
Causes of hypovolaemia and hypervolaemia

Hypovolaemia
  Gastrointestinal sodium loss
    e.g. vomiting, diarrhoea, nasogastric suction
  Skin sodium loss
    e.g. excessive sweating, burns
  Renal sodium loss
    e.g. diuretics, mineralocorticoid deficiency,
      tubulointerstitial disease
  Internal sequestration
    e.g. bowel obstruction, peritonitis, pancreatitis, crush
      injury
  Haemorrhage

Hypervolaemia
  Iatrogenic
    e.g. salt loading (oral or intravenous)
  Renal sodium retention in generalized oedema states
    e.g. congestive cardiac failure, cirrhosis, nephrotic
      syndrome
  Renal sodium retention in renal failure
    e.g. acute and chronic renal failure (usual case)
  Renal sodium retention in primary mineralocorticoid excess
    e.g. Conn's syndrome (note no oedema)

Glomerular filtration

Glomerular filtration is the process whereby a clear fluid, from which blood cells and macromolecules such as proteins are excluded, is produced from the blood perfusing the glomerulus at the beginning of each nephron. This ultrafiltration process, which occurs largely as a result of the hydrostatic pressure in the arterial tree generated by the heart, is described in more detail in Chapter 5. The ultrafiltrate so produced contains electrolytes and small solutes in plasma-like concentrations, and constitutes the 'primary' urine from which the final excreted urine is derived.

Tubular modification

This step involves the alteration of the volume and composition of the glomerular filtrate by transport processes carried out along the length of the tubular system. The dominant modification overall is the reabsorption of the great majority (over 99%) of the filtered fluid, together with most of its solute content (notably sodium). However, some electrolytes and many 'foreign' organic molecules undergo transport *into* the tubular fluid, a process called secretion. The final urine excreted from the kidneys reflects the net effect of all these tubular transport processes.

It is important to note in Fig. 2.4 that not all of the blood plasma brought to the nephron is filtered at the glomerulus. Of the plasma flow delivered to each nephron, some 20% becomes glomerular filtrate while the remaining 80% emerges from the glomerulus and is carried by postglomerular capillaries around the tubular structures of that (and adjacent) nephrons, where it is available for transport exchanges with the luminal fluid. The ratio of the glomerular filtration rate (GFR) to the renal plasma flow (RPF) is called the filtration fraction (FF), and is about 0.2 in man.

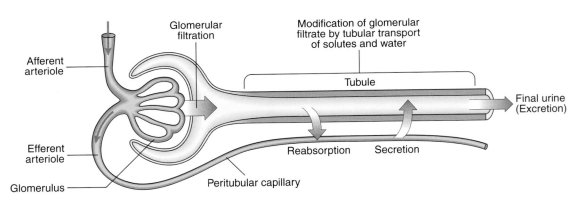

Fig. 2.4
Functional anatomy of the nephron.

Some approximate figures will serve to illustrate the relative magnitude of these processes. The kidneys receive about one-fifth of the cardiac output, which for an adult woman like Joanne may be 4.5 L/min. Thus the total renal blood flow (RBF) would be 900 mL/min. Assuming a haematocrit (red blood cell volume as a fraction of total blood volume) of 0.45, the RPF would be almost 500 mL/min (i.e. $(1 - 0.45) \times 900$). If the filtration fraction is 0.2, her GFR will be 100 mL/min. Given 99% reabsorption of the filtrate volume, this corresponds to a typical urine flow rate of 1 mL/min. On a daily basis, the corresponding figures are a GFR of 144 litres/24 h, and a daily urine output of 1.4 litres/24 h.

Nephron segments

A more anatomically detailed view of the tubular structures comprising the nephron is given in Fig. 2.5. Each of the kidney's one million nephrons has its glomerulus located in the renal cortex (see Chapter 1). Blood is delivered through a series of branches of the renal artery until it enters each glomerulus via an afferent arteriole. After breaking up into the capillary loops

constituting the glomerulus, the blood emerges via an efferent arteriole which itself gives rise to the network of peritubular capillaries. These eventually join to take the blood away from the kidney via the renal vein. (The vascular structures are shown in more detail in Fig. 1.2.)

The segments of the tubular system attached to each glomerulus are named, in order, the proximal tubule, the loop of Henle, the distal tubule and the collecting duct. Each segment consists of specialized epithelial cells adapted to perform particular transport functions.

The proximal tubule is some 2–3 mm long. It forms a number of turns, or convolutions, before descending in a straight segment (pars recta) down into the outer medulla. Its cells are characterized by a prominent brush border consisting of numerous elongated processes arising from the apical (lumen-facing) cell membrane. Many mitochondria lie between the extensive invaginations of the basolateral (blood-facing) membrane.

The loop of Henle descends from the outer medulla a variable distance into the inner medulla, going deepest for loops arising from nephrons having their glomeruli located in the inner cortex (the juxtamedullary nephrons). It consists of a thin descending limb and, after a hairpin turn, a shorter thin ascending segment, both of which comprise flat cells with few mitochondria and little membrane amplification. The cells of the thick ascending limb, on the other hand, are larger and contain abundant mitochondria and extensive basolateral infoldings, suggestive of a role in active ion transport.

The distal tubule starts within the cortex at the point where the thick ascending limb passes by the glomerulus of the related nephron, where it forms the macula densa (see later in this chapter). The early part of the distal segment is convoluted, with metabolically active cells. The later part is straight, and joins with similar segments from adjacent nephrons to form the cortical collecting duct, with which it has structural and functional similarities (and indeed a common embryological origin from the ureteric bud; see Fig. 1.3).

The medullary collecting duct arises in continuity with the cortical collecting duct as it crosses the corticomedullary junction. The lumen becomes progressively wider as it passes towards the tip of the renal papilla, where it empties into the calyces and the renal pelvis.

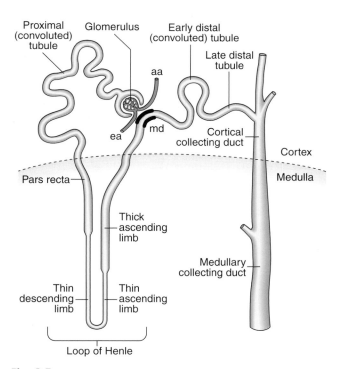

Fig. 2.5
Microscopic structure of the nephron, showing names of successive tubular segments. aa, afferent arteriole; ea, efferent arteriole; md, macula densa. (Refer to Fig. 1.2 for details of vascular elements.)

Sodium transport

An appreciation of the mechanisms involved in handling sodium in the nephron is of crucial importance in understanding how our patient's body fluid depletion has come about. As mentioned previously, over 99% of the fluid filtered is normally reabsorbed along the tubular system of the nephron, and this is largely related to the reabsorption of a similar proportion of filtered sodium. Assuming a plasma Na concentration of 140 mmol/L and a GFR of 144 L/day, the amount of sodium passed into the filtrate is 140 × 144, which equals 20 160 mmol/day. For a person consuming some 100 mmol of sodium per day in the diet, daily balance with regard to sodium requires the excretion of 100 mmol Na/day into the final urine (neglecting the very small losses through the gut and skin). This represents just (100/20 160) or 0.5% of the sodium contained in the glomerular filtrate, so we conclude that 99.5% of the filtered sodium load must be reabsorbed by the tubules.

The segments in which this reabsorptive activity occurs have been defined by micropuncture experiments in animal models. Microscopic amounts of fluid are sampled from different points along the nephron, and their composition is compared to that of the filtered fluid. Table 2.3 shows the estimated contributions by successive tubular segments under normal conditions which have been deduced by these experiments.

In the following sections, an outline of the cellular mechanism of sodium reabsorption in each of these segments will be provided.

Proximal tubule

Much of the cortical tissue mass in the kidney consists of proximal tubules, and these are the most metabolically active cells in the kidney. This activity is directed primarily towards the reabsorption of some two-thirds (nearly 70%) of the sodium contained in the glomerular filtrate, together with associated solutes and water.

The mechanisms involved in this reabsorptive process are complex, and will only be outlined here.

The following are some transport properties of the proximal tubule:

- The process occurs almost isotonically, i.e. the osmolality of the tubular fluid falls only very slightly below that of the plasma along the length of the tubule.
- Sodium reabsorption is associated with complete reabsorption of filtered glucose and amino acids (when plasma concentrations are normal), and almost complete reabsorption of bicarbonate and phosphate ions.
- Reabsorption of all solutes and water is very sensitive to metabolic poisons.
- There is a very high water permeability across the proximal tubular cell layer.
- There is a low electrical potential difference across the tubular epithelial wall.

From these and other detailed observations, a model for the operation of a typical cell in this tubular segment has been developed, as shown in Fig. 2.6.

The primary active transport step underlying absorption of sodium and, secondarily, other solutes and water, is the Na,K-dependent ATPase located along the basolateral (blood-facing) membrane of the proximal tubular cells. This pump lowers the sodium concentration inside the cell to around 5–10 mmol/L, thereby creating a marked electrochemical gradient for the entry of sodium from the tubular fluid (where it is

Table 2.3
Sodium reabsorption in successive segments of the nephron

Tubular segment	Sodium reabsorption
Proximal tubule	65%
Loop of Henle (thick ascending limb)	25%
Distal tubule	
Early (convoluted segment)	6%
Late (initial/cortical collecting duct)	2–3%
Medullary collecting duct	< 1%

Amounts reabsorbed at each site are expressed as a percentage of the filtered load of sodium.

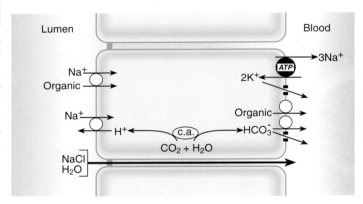

Fig. 2.6
Principal transport properties of a proximal tubule cell. Open circles represent carrier molecules without direct linkage to ATP hydrolysis; blackened circles are carriers with such linkage (primary active transport pumps). Gaps in cell membranes represent ion channels. c.a., carbonic anhydrase. The arrow between cells indicates the paracellular shunt pathway. Note that the potassium ions taken up by the basolateral sodium–potassium pump 'recycle' across that membrane via a potassium channel.

present in plasma-like concentrations) across the apical cell membrane into the cell. Located in this membrane are several carrier proteins through which sodium entry is coupled with the transport of other solutes, which themselves move against their electrochemical gradient (or 'uphill') by what is termed secondary active transport.

Two types of such carriers are particularly important. One group mediates the cotransport of a variety of organic solutes from the luminal fluid in conjunction with sodium. In this group are a number of carrier molecules, each with specificity for a different substance, e.g. a sodium–glucose cotransporter, a family of related sodium–amino acid cotransporters, a sodium–phosphate cotransporter, and so on.

A second carrier type mediates the countertransport of an absorbed sodium ion with a hydrogen ion produced within the epithelial cell. This sodium–hydrogen exchanger (NHE-3) is one of a family of such proteins having widespread ramifications for cellular acid–base metabolism, and is important in the mechanism of proximal bicarbonate reabsorption (see Chapter 4).

While these and other mechanisms for the movement of sodium into the proximal tubular cells from the luminal fluid are well documented, they can account for only a fraction of the total reabsorptive flux of sodium which occurs across the epithelium. More than half of this sodium movement appears to occur between adjacent epithelial cells, through what is termed the 'shunt' pathway. A component of this flux is driven by transepithelial electrical gradients, but some sodium and other ions are carried across the tubular wall by 'solvent drag', pulled in the bulk flow of water which is known to occur through the intercellular pathway. This water flux itself is driven partly by the small but significant osmotic (and oncotic) gradients established across the proximal tubular wall along its length, and partly by a small hydrostatic pressure gradient favouring fluid movement from the tubular lumen into the peritubular capillaries.

Loop of Henle

The cells of the thin descending limb of the loop of Henle do not carry out active transepithelial ion transport, but act as important passive equilibrators in the process of countercurrent multiplication (see Chapter 3). The thick ascending limb segment, on the other hand, is responsible for reabsorption of a further 25% of the filtered load of sodium, and contributes importantly to the build-up of the medullary interstitial concentration gradient which is essential in the

mechanism for ultimate concentration of the urine (see Chapter 3).

The transport properties of the thick ascending limb include the following:

- Extensive transepithelial reabsorption of sodium and chloride is accompanied by smaller fluxes of potassium, magnesium and calcium.
- This nephron segment is impermeable to water under all conditions.
- Transport of all ions across this segment is powerfully inhibited by loop-acting diuretic drugs such as furosemide (frusemide).
- A small lumen-positive transepithelial potential difference normally exists across this segment.

Studies of the mechanism of ion transport in the thick ascending limb have given rise to the cell model shown in Fig. 2.7. As in the proximal tubule, the primary active transport step is the Na,K-ATPase located on the basolateral cell membrane. In this cell, however, sodium entry from the luminal fluid across the apical cell membrane is via a quite different mechanism than that operating in the proximal tubule. Here, one sodium ion, one potassium ion and two chloride ions interact with a carrier protein molecule embedded in the apical cell membrane ('the triple cotransporter', or NKCCT). It is this carrier whose function is blocked by loop diuretics such as furosemide (frusemide), which therefore results in the inhibition of the reabsorptive activity of this segment. Note that the movement of sodium into the cell via this carrier is electrochemically 'downhill', but is coupled through the action of the carrier to the uphill transport

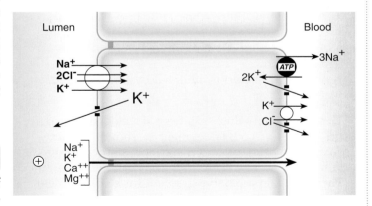

Fig. 2.7

Principal transport properties of a cell in the thick ascending limb of the loop of Henle. The ⊕ indicates that the transepithelial electrical potential difference is positive in the lumen relative to the blood side. Symbol conventions as in Fig. 2.6. See text for detailed description.

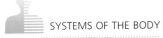
of chloride and potassium. Of the potassium accumulated inside the cell, some is transported out of the cell across the basolateral membrane, in part coupled with chloride, resulting in net reabsorption of potassium across the epithelium. However, a component of intracellular potassium recycles through a potassium channel in the apical cell membrane into the lumen, where it becomes available for re-entry into the cell through the triple cotransporter. It should be noted that there is considerable flux of cations such as sodium, potassium, calcium and magnesium across this epithelium via the shunt pathway between adjacent cells, driven largely by the lumen-positive transepithelial potential difference.

The fact that this tubular segment is impermeable to water under all conditions means that it acts as a site of dilution of the luminal fluid, i.e. removal of electrolytes but not water lowers the luminal osmolality. At the same time, however, the segment plays a vital role in building the concentrating capacity of the renal medulla, as will be explained in the next chapter. It is therefore a critical portion of the nephron not only for net electrolyte reabsorption, but in contributing to the regulation of the osmolality of the body fluids. All of these processes are disrupted by agents such as loop diuretics which interfere with the operation of this segment.

Distal tubule

The transport properties of the early distal tubule (or distal convoluted tubule) include the following:

- Sodium is reabsorbed with chloride but with little net potassium movement.
- Water permeability is very low under all conditions.
- A further component of filtered calcium is reabsorbed.
- Sodium transport is inhibited by thiazides and related drugs.

The cell model which has been developed to explain the operation of this segment is shown in Fig. 2.8. Again, the primary active transport step is the operation of the Na,K-ATPase in the basolateral membrane. There is again a passive gradient for sodium to enter the cell from the luminal fluid across the apical cell membrane, and in this segment this uptake step is mediated by a sodium–chloride cotransport carrier molecule (called the NCT), in which one sodium and one chloride ion are taken up simultaneously. It is this carrier whose function is blocked by the thiazide diuretics and related molecules, resulting in the loss of unreabsorbed sodium chloride into the urine.

While no significant potassium fluxes occur across this cell segment, transepithelial calcium reabsorption does occur by the mechanisms shown in Fig. 2.8. This involves uptake of calcium across the apical cell membrane via a calcium channel, with extrusion of calcium across the basolateral membrane via a sodium–calcium countertransport carrier, driven by the passive inward movement of sodium from the ECF. Thus, during thiazide action, sodium entry into the cell is inhibited, resulting in a lowering of intracellular sodium by the continued action of the basolateral Na,K-ATPase. This in turn increases the activity of the basal sodium–calcium exchanger, resulting in lower cell calcium and an enhanced entry of calcium through the apical membrane, and hence across the epithelium. This explains the apparent paradox of treatment with thiazide diuretics in which sodium excretion is increased but calcium excretion is decreased.

Cortical collecting duct

The late segment of the distal tubule has similar transport properties to the earliest part of the collecting duct system, formed where two distal tubular segments join together. These properties continue until the collecting duct leaves the cortex to become the medullary collecting duct.

The transport properties of this nephron segment include the following:

- There is reabsorption of some 2–3% of the filtered sodium load, accompanied in part by chloride reabsorption, potassium secretion and acid secretion into the lumen.

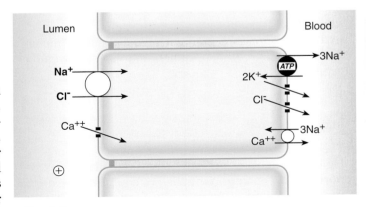

Fig. 2.8
Principal transport properties of an early distal tubule (distal convoluted tubule) cell. Symbol conventions as in Fig. 2.6. See text for detailed description. The lumen is electrically positive with respect to the blood side.

- All of these transport processes are stimulated by the circulating steroid hormone aldosterone.
- Water permeability of this segment is variable, being increased by circulating antidiuretic hormone (vasopressin).
- Sodium reabsorption in this segment is inhibited by amiloride and (when aldosterone is acting) spironolactone; when these drugs are present, secretion of both K^+ and H^+ is reduced.
- There is normally an appreciable lumen-negative transepithelial potential difference, but this is largely abolished by the action of amiloride and spironolactone.

The cell mechanisms which have been proposed to account for these transport properties are shown in Fig. 2.9. There are two distinct cell types defined histologically in this segment, mediating different transport functions.

The principal cells are the site of sodium reabsorption and potassium secretion. Again the primary active transport step driving these processes is the basolateral Na,K-ATPase. Sodium enters the cell from the luminal fluid down its electrochemical gradient, passing in this instance through a channel called the epithelial sodium channel, or ENaC. This step generates a lumen-negative diffusion potential. Potassium accumulated in the cell moves into the luminal fluid through an apical potassium channel, down its electrochemical gradient. This cell type is also known to be a target for the action of aldosterone, which enters the cell from the blood, and interacts with a receptor molecule located in the cytoplasm. The hormone–receptor complex undergoes translocation into the nucleus, after which transcription and translation of aldosterone-induced proteins occurs, resulting in activation of all the transport steps undertaken by this cell. In addition, this cell contains basolateral membrane receptors for circulating vasopressin, the action of which results in increased transepithelial water transport in this segment (see also Chapter 3).

The intercalated cells are the site of acid secretion into the lumen within this tubular segment. This is mediated by an active hydrogen pump, the H^+-ATPase, located on the apical cell membrane, which translocates hydrogen ions from the cell cytoplasm into the lumen. These hydrogen ions are generated within the cell by the action of carbonic anhydrase, which catalyses the formation of carbonic acid from water and carbon dioxide. This disassociates into a hydrogen ion which is secreted into the lumen and a bicarbonate ion which enters the ECF across the basolateral membrane, partly in exchange for chloride via an anion countertransporter. This process of acid secretion is also activated by aldosterone.

This nephron segment is sensitive to a number of transport inhibitors. Amiloride blocks the apical sodium channel in the principal cells. This results not only in inhibition of sodium reabsorption, but also greatly reduces potassium and acid secretion, which are partly dependent on the negative lumen potential generated by sodium reabsorption. Spironolactone blocks the binding of aldosterone to its cytoplasmic receptor, thereby interfering with the activation by aldosterone of sodium reabsorption, potassium secretion and acid secretion.

It should be mentioned that, under unusual metabolic conditions, namely potassium depletion and alkalosis, this nephron segment is able to adapt its transport functions to mediate potassium reabsorption and bicarbonate secretion (respectively), though these processes are not active under normal dietary and metabolic conditions.

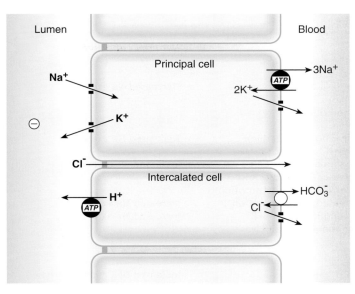

Fig. 2.9
Principal transport properties of the cells of the late distal tubule/cortical collecting duct. Symbol conventions as in Fig. 2.6. See text for detailed description. The lumen is electrically negative with respect to the blood side.

Regulation of sodium transport

A number of mechanisms interact to ensure that sodium excretion by the kidney is appropriately matched to changes in sodium intake and the ECF volume. These mechanisms require the precisely balanced operation of various sensory systems which detect changes in the ECF volume (and related parameters), and a number of effector mechanisms capable of altering the kidney's sodium excretion rate.

The sensing mechanisms include:

- Volume receptors in the cardiac atria and intrathoracic veins.
- Pressure receptors in the central arterial tree and the afferent arterioles within the kidney.
- Tubular fluid NaCl concentration receptors within the distal nephron (the macula densa).

The intrathoracic volume receptors respond to reduced distension by signalling to the brainstem that central venous volume has fallen, resulting in activation of effector mechanisms to restore the volume and pressure within the circulation. The opposite responses take place during ECF volume expansion. In addition, during volume expansion increased stretch of the cardiac atria directly results in the release of atrial natriuretic peptide (see below). Other afferents arise from arterial basoreceptors in the aortic arch and carotid sinus and these give signals paralleling those of the volume receptors in most circumstances. The operation of the intrarenal baroreceptors and the macula densa is explained below in the section on the renin–angiotensin–aldosterone system.

The effector mechanisms involved in adjusting renal sodium excretion are summarized in Table 2.4.

Of the neurohumoral mechanisms, the most important is the renin–angiotensin–aldosterone (RAA)

system. As illustrated in Fig. 2.10, this system is activated by stimuli leading to the release of renin, an enzyme contained within specialized smooth muscle cells in the walls of the afferent and efferent arterioles. The principal stimuli to its release are as follows:

- Reduced perfusion pressure in the afferent arteriole.
- Increased sympathetic nerve activity in fibres innervating the afferent and efferent arterioles.
- Decreased sodium chloride concentration flowing through the distal tubule.

The inset in Fig. 2.10 shows the anatomical arrangements whereby the afferent and efferent arterioles of a given nephron come into direct contact with the earliest part of that nephron's distal tubule, where the epithelial cells become modified to form the macula densa. This juxtaglomerular apparatus brings together the three principal stimuli promoting renin release: thus when ECF volume is low, the pressure distending the afferent arteriole falls, sympathetic nerve discharges to the renin-containing cells increase, and sodium concentration in the distal tubular lumen falls because of activated sodium reabsorption in earlier tubular segments.

The renin released into the circulation acts to cleave the peptide substrate angiotensinogen (manufactured in the liver), producing angiotensin I in the circulation. After passage through capillary beds, notably in the

Table 2.4
Effector mechanisms involved in regulation of renal sodium transport

Effector system	Site of action	Net effect of activation
Neurohumoral mechanisms		
Renin–angiotensin–aldosterone system	PT (angiotensin II), causing increased Na reabsorption	Decreased Na excretion
	CCD (aldosterone), causing increased Na reabsorption	
Sympathetic nervous system/catecholamines	PT (noradrenaline; norepinephrine), causing increased Na reabsorption	Decreased Na excretion
Atrial natriuretic peptide	Glomerulus, causing increased GFR	Increased Na excretion
	PT, causing decreased Na reabsorption	
	MCD, causing decreased Na reabsorption	
Natriuretic hormone	PT, causing decreased Na reabsorption	Increased Na excretion
Prostaglandins	Glomerulus, causing increased GFR	Increased Na excretion
	TAL and CCD, causing decreased Na reabsorption	
Haemodynamic-mechanical mechanisms		
GFR changes	Glomerulus	Increased GFR causes increased Na excretion
Peritubular physical forces (hydrostatic and oncotic pressures in the peritubular capillaries)	PT	Increased filtration fraction causes decreased Na excretion

Note that the table excludes a number of mediators of altered sodium transport whose physiological role is not well established. PT, proximal tubule; CCD, cortical collecting duct (including late distal tubules forming initial collecting duct); TAL, thick ascending limb of the loop of Henle; MCD, medullary collecting duct; GFR, glomerular filtration rate.

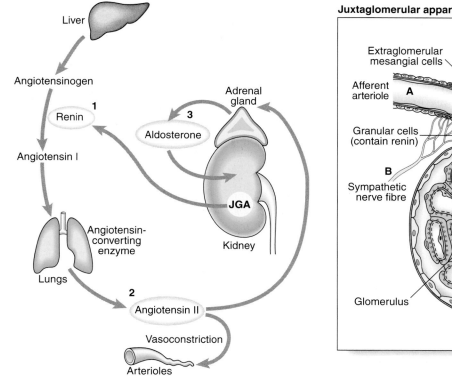

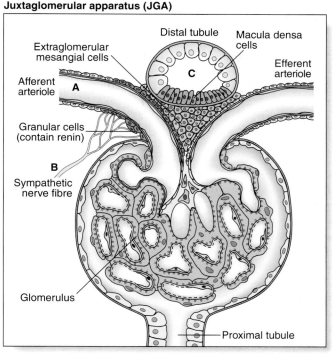

Juxtaglomerular apparatus (JGA)

Fig. 2.10

The renin–angiotensin–aldosterone system. The numbers 1–3 show the sequence of steps in the activation of the system. The inset shows the juxtaglomerular apparatus (JGA) with major stimuli acting as triggers for renin release: A, fall in pressure in afferent arteriole; B, release of noradrenaline (norepinephrine) by sympathetic nerve endings on granular cells; C, fall in NaCl concentration in distal tubule. Note that angiotensin II has a number of additional actions not shown on this figure (see text).

lungs, this is cleaved by angiotensin-converting enzyme into angiotensin II. This octapeptide is the central mediator of the RAA system, having multiple actions:

- It directly acts to vasoconstrict small arterioles.
- It directly stimulates proximal tubular sodium reabsorption.
- It causes the zona glomerulosa cells of the adrenal cortex to release the steroid hormone aldosterone.

As described earlier in this chapter, aldosterone acts to stimulate salt reabsorption in the cortical collecting duct of the nephron, hence reducing sodium and water excretion from the kidney. The net effect of these actions is to restore blood pressure and ECF volume towards normal, thereby decreasing the stimulus which led to the activation of the system.

The sympathetic nervous system is also involved in the response to hypovolaemia, not only by acting as a stimulus for renin release, described above, but also by releasing noradrenaline (norepinephrine) around the proximal tubular cells, where it directly stimulates tubular sodium reabsorption. In addition, sympathetic activation vasoconstricts the afferent arteriole, reducing GFR and further limiting sodium and fluid losses.

Most of the other humoral mechanisms involved in sodium regulation lead to an increase in sodium excretion, thereby playing an important role in defending against volume expansion during periods of high salt availability.

Atrial natriuretic peptide is released from the cardiac atria when they undergo stretch during high volume states. It circulates as a peptide containing 28 amino acids and has numerous actions contributing to enhanced sodium excretion:

- The GFR is increased, via an action of atrial natriuretic peptide to dilate the afferent arterioles.
- Sodium reabsorption by the proximal tubule and medullary collecting duct is inhibited.
- Secretion of renin and aldosterone is reduced, further switching off sodium-retaining systems.

A less well defined mediator of sodium excretion during volume expansion is the natriuretic hormone released from the brain during these conditions. It is known to have ouabain- or digoxin-like properties in that it inhibits Na,K-ATPase in both vascular smooth muscle and renal epithelial cells. In the former, the result is an increase in intracellular sodium and calcium concentrations leading to vasoconstriction, while in the kidney the effect is an inhibition of sodium reabsorption, promoting natriuresis (increased sodium excretion).

A variety of other intrarenal mediators are involved in inhibiting sodium reabsorption under certain physiological conditions, and of these the most important clinically is the intrarenal prostaglandin (PG) system. Locally acting prostaglandins, PGE_2 in particular, are known to enhance glomerular filtration and decrease sodium reabsorption in the thick ascending limb of the loop of Henle and in the cortical collecting duct, the net effect being enhancement of sodium excretion. Other systems which have been implicated in sodium transport regulation include dopamine, kinins, nitric oxide and endothelin. The role of these mediators under physiological conditions is incompletely defined at the present time.

Another important system involved in the response to major (5–10%) changes in circulating volume is antidiuretic hormone. This effector peptide acts both to increase water reabsorption from the nephron and to vasoconstrict blood vessels, with little direct effect on sodium balance. It will be described in more detail in Chapter 3.

Haemodynamic and mechanical mechanisms are also involved in the maintenance of sodium balance. Changes in GFR are involved in mediating the actions of some of the neurohumoral mechanisms outlined above. Minor minute-to-minute changes in GFR are usually not a determinant of sodium excretion, largely because of the phenomenon of glomerulotubular balance: this describes the proportional adjustment of proximal reabsorption to shifts in GFR, minimizing the net excretory effect of such changes. During wider swings in circulating blood volume, proximal tubular reabsorption is thought to be altered by changes in the physical forces affecting sodium and fluid reabsorption from the proximal tubule, namely the hydrostatic and oncotic pressures in the peritubular capillaries.

See box 3.

Looking first at Joanne's urea, creatinine and urate results, we note that the urea and urate are elevated, while the creatinine is within the normal range. As will be discussed further in Chapter 5, creatinine acts as a marker of the GFR, and the fact that it is not significantly elevated suggests that the GFR has not fallen greatly (though a small rise in creatinine within the normal range cannot be excluded). The increase in

---

Body fluids and nephron function box 3

Biochemistry results

We can now understand that Joanne's symptoms and signs of volume depletion have resulted from the action of the furosemide (frusemide) tablets she had been taking, resulting in inhibition of sodium reabsorption in the loop of Henle, and hence negative net sodium balance.

Further investigation included the following biochemistry results:

Sodium 136 mmol/L
*Potassium 2.7 mmol/L
Chloride 95 mmol/L
*Bicarbonate 32 mmol/L
*Urea 10.5 mmol/L
Creatinine 0.12 mmol/L
*Urate 0.48 mmol/L.

These results lead us to the following question:

How have the abnormalities in her biochemical profile come about?

(*Results outside the normal range; see Appendix.)

---

plasma urea is consistent with hypovolaemia, since urea is handled by the kidney both by filtration and by partial reabsorption within the nephron, the extent of which is increased during low volume states (a number of other factors can influence the plasma urea, as described in Chapter 5).

The increase in plasma urate (the anion base of uric acid) is also suggestive of volume depletion. This nitrogenous breakdown product of nucleic acid metabolism is freely filtered at the glomerulus, but undergoes both extensive reabsorption from and secretion into the proximal tubule, usually resulting in a final excretion of some 10% of the filtered urate load. However, during volume contraction, the forces promoting increased proximal tubular sodium and fluid reabsorption also increase the absorptive component of proximal urate transport, resulting in elevated plasma urate concentration. Indeed, in susceptible individuals, this can result in an attack of gout because of uric acid crystallization in joint tissues and the resulting inflammation.

Joanne's electrolyte results show that the sodium and chloride concentrations are normal, while the potassium concentration is reduced and the bicarbonate concentration elevated. It is important to recognize that the normal sodium concentration does not reflect a normal total body sodium, as indeed we have concluded that she has been partly depleted of sodium because of the action of the diuretic. The normal concentration simply reflects the fact that water loss from the ECF has been roughly proportionate to sodium, resulting in no net change in the ECF sodium concentration or osmolality. (Disturbances of sodium concentration may be seen during diuretic treatment under certain conditions, as discussed in the next chapter.)

To understand the origin of the hypokalaemia, we need to review mechanisms regulating potassium balance.

Potassium transport

Potassium is freely filtered at the glomerulus and, like sodium, some 65% of the filtered amount is reabsorbed in the proximal tubule. Again paralleling sodium, about 25% more is reabsorbed in the thick ascending limb of the loop of Henle. While no potassium is transported in the early (convoluted) distal tubule, in the late distal tubule joining the cortical collecting duct potassium is actually transported into the tubular fluid by a process of secretion. This secretory step is carried out by the mechanisms illustrated in Fig. 2.9 – the principal cell of the cortical collecting duct.

Under conditions of low potassium intake, the extent of secretion may be minimal, resulting in a net fractional excretion of potassium of some 10% of the filtered load. During potassium depletion, net reabsorption from the cortical and medullary collecting duct can even occur, resulting in fractional excretion rates as low as 5%. More commonly, however, under normal dietary conditions or during potassium loading, potassium secretion can be stimulated such that the final urine contains 20% or more of the filtered potassium amount.

The factors regulating the extent of potassium secretion in the cortical collecting duct segment include:

- Circulating factors
  - high plasma aldosterone concentration
  - high plasma potassium concentration
  - high plasma pH.
- Luminal factors
  - high sodium delivery rate
  - high luminal flow rate
  - negative lumen potential difference.

Aldosterone acts as the key regulator of potassium balance, in parallel with its role in sodium metabolism but mediated by a quite different feedback mechanism. As shown in Fig. 2.11, a high plasma potassium concentration resulting from increased dietary potassium or other reasons directly stimulates the zona glomerulosa cells of the adrenal cortex to secrete aldosterone, which, by increasing potassium secretion into the

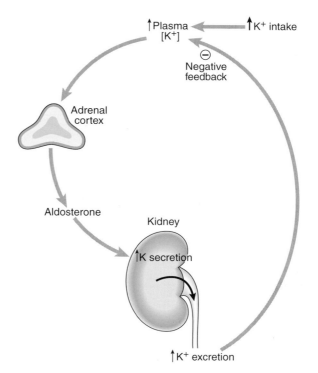

Fig. 2.11
Feedback control of the plasma potassium concentration.

distal nephron, leads to increased potassium excretion, thereby reducing the high plasma potassium. This is the main negative feedback mechanism responsible for maintaining the plasma potassium within the range 3.5–5.0 mmol/L.

Of the luminal factors, the rate of delivery of sodium and fluid from the earlier nephron segments is an important determinant of potassium secretion because of their influence on the transport processes of the cortical collecting duct.

From the above, it can be seen why a diuretic drug acting to inhibit loop of Henle sodium reabsorption would lead to potassium depletion. The following factors may be involved:

- The potassium normally reabsorbed across the thick ascending limb is lost into the urine.
- The sodium not reabsorbed in the loop passes through to the distal tubule and cortical collecting duct where it is available for increased exchange for potassium through the principal cell mechanisms.
- The increased flow of fluid accompanying sodium through the distal potassium-secretory segment dilutes the luminal fluid and so provides an increased gradient for potassium to move into the lumen.

- The volume depletion resulting from diuretic action stimulates aldosterone (via renin and angiotensin), further amplifying potassium secretion.

Hypokalaemia can be caused by a variety of other disturbances, as shown in Table 2.5. Note that in some cases the low ECF potassium concentration results largely from a shift into the larger ICF pool. When external losses do occur, this may be from either the gastrointestinal tract or the kidney. Frequently, losses occur from both systems since, when there is a reduction in ECF volume, aldosterone promotes potassium secretion in the kidney and hence increases urinary potassium excretion.

Table 2.5
Causes of hypokalaemia

Redistribution into cells
  e.g. alkalosis, catecholamines, insulin excess, hypokalaemic periodic paralysis
Inadequate K intake
  e.g. starvation, inadequate replacement after operation
Increased external K losses
  gastrointestinal tract
    e.g. vomiting, diarrhoea, laxative abuse, villous adenoma of rectum
  kidney
    e.g. high mineralocorticoid activity (hyperaldosteronism, steroid therapy, etc.), diuretics, classic (distal) renal tubular acidosis, congenital tubular transport disorders

The increase in plasma bicarbonate in Joanne's case reflects a mild metabolic alkalosis, largely owing to the enhancement of hydrogen ion secretion resulting from increased sodium delivery through the cortical collecting duct segment, as outlined above. Again, enhancement of this step by high levels of aldosterone serves to aggravate this loss of acid.

Pharmacology of diuretic agents

This chapter has introduced the mechanisms of action of a number of commonly used diuretic drugs. For completion, a summary of the major agents in clinical use, together with their principal properties and actions, is given in Tables 2.6 and 2.7.

An important generalization about most of the drugs used as diuretics is that they act on the mechanism for sodium uptake from the luminal fluid across the apical cell membrane in a particular tubular segment. This gives rise to the specificity of their site of action, given that the apical uptake step is mediated by different mechanisms in each segment, as described earlier. In contrast, the sodium exit step from the base of the cells is the same in each tubular segment, namely the Na,K-ATPase step.

One group of diuretic drugs not shown in the accompanying tables is the osmotic diuretics. These substances are freely filtered but are not reabsorbed

Table 2.6
Summary of sites and mechanisms of action of the principal classes of diuretic drugs

Site	Drug class	Prototype drug	Mechanism of action
Proximal tubule	Carbonic anhydrase inhibitors	Acetazolamide	Prevent $NaHCO_3$ reabsorption by limiting H^+ formation
Thick ascending limb of loop of Henle	'Loop' diuretics	Furosemide (frusemide)	Block apical Na, K, 2Cl cotransporter
Early distal tubule	Thiazides and related drugs	Chlorothiazide	Block apical Na, Cl cotransporter
Late distal tubule/cortical collecting duct	a. Sodium channel blockers b. Aldosterone antagonists	a. Amiloride b. Spironolactone	a. Block apical Na channel b. Block aldosterone receptor in cytoplasm

Table 2.7
Effects of diuretics on renal electrolyte and water excretion

Diuretic class	Na excretion*	K excretion	Anion excreted	Concentrating capacity[†]	Diluting capacity[†]
Carbonic anhydrase inhibitors	5	Increased	HCO_3^-	Increased	Increased
Loop blockers	20	Increased	Cl^-	Decreased	Decreased
Thiazides	6	Increased	Cl^-	No change	Decreased
K-sparing drugs	2	Decreased	Cl^-/HCO_3^-	No change	No change

*Maximum percentage of filtered load of Na excreted into the urine during diuretic action. [†] Effect of the diuretic on the capacity of the kidney to concentrate and dilute the urine (see Chapter 3).

by any part of the tubular system. Their action is thus not site-specific in that they entrain fluid osmotically within the tubular lumen and therefore limit the extent of sodium reabsorption in multiple segments. The principal clinical example of such an agent is mannitol, which must be given by intravenous infusion, and is used to achieve short-term diuresis in conditions associated with cell swelling, such as cerebral oedema.

All the other diuretic drugs detailed in the tables (except spironolactone) must be delivered into the luminal fluid in appreciable concentrations to affect the apical sodium transport mechanisms. Delivery to the site of action is achieved partly by filtration, but there is an important component of active secretion of the diuretic molecules across the proximal tubular epithelium, mediated by the transport mechanisms available to secrete weak organic acids and bases in this nephron segment. This is of particular importance in determining the pharmacokinetics of these drugs since most are strongly protein-bound in the plasma, a property which itself leads to a very low delivery rate into the tubule by glomerular filtration alone.

More background information concerning the action of carbonic anhydrase inhibitors and the effects of diuretics on concentrating and diluting capacity is given in the subsequent two chapters of this volume.

Clinical use of diuretics

The two commonest indications for diuretic prescription are in the treatment of hypertension (see Chapter 9) and in the reduction of ECF volume in oedematous states (see Chapter 6).

Diuretic use is frequently complicated by a number of adverse effects, which are summarized in Table 2.8. These fall broadly into three categories: physiologically predictable side effects (including abnormal plasma electrolyte concentrations), metabolic side effects (including effects on glucose and lipid metabolism, where the mechanism is poorly defined), and allergic or idiosyncratic reactions. The latter are most prominent with drugs in the sulphonamide class, including carbonic anhydrase inhibitors, furosemide (frusemide) and the thiazides.

There are a number of indications for the rational prescription of combinations of diuretic drugs. First, to reduce an unwanted electrolyte effect such as hypokalaemia induced by one class of agents (loop and early distal drugs), simultaneous treatment with a potassium-sparing drug such as amiloride can lead to a more neutral net effect on potassium balance while

Table 2.8
Adverse effects of diuretic drug use

'Physiological' side effects
  Hypovolaemia
  Hyponatraemia
  Hypokalaemia*
  Metabolic alkalosis*
  Hyperuricaemia
  Hypomagnesaemia*
  Hypocalcaemia (loop-acting drugs only)
Metabolic side effects
  Glucose intolerance/hyperglycaemia
  Hyperlipidaemia
Miscellaneous side effects
  Hypersensitivity reactions
  Acute pancreatitis/cholecystitis (thiazides)
  Impotence

The effects shown apply chiefly to the loop and early distal acting drugs.
*These effects are not seen with drugs acting in the cortical collecting duct; these may cause the opposite side effects (hyperkalaemia and metabolic acidosis). Carbonic anhydrase inhibitors may cause hypokalaemia with metabolic acidosis.

maintaining adequate diuretic action. Second, in resistant oedema associated with advanced disease of the heart or kidneys, it is sometimes appropriate to coadminister drugs acting at multiple sites along the nephron to counter the 'resistance' which may develop to one agent because of compensatory enhancement of sodium reabsorption by more distally located segments. In these circumstances the prescriber must take particular care to avoid complications resulting from uncontrolled losses of fluid and electrolytes by careful clinical and laboratory monitoring.

In general, the following summarizes the guidelines for diuretic use under most conditions:

- Use the minimum effective dose.
- Use for as short a period of time as necessary.
- Monitor regularly for adverse effects.
- Use only for appropriate indications.

In regard to the last point, Joanne's use of diuretics for cosmetic or weight control purposes is clearly inappropriate.

Principles of fluid and electrolyte replacement therapy

The key steps in correcting a disturbance in body fluid and electrolyte composition are:

1. Cessation or reversal of the causative disturbance.
2. Replacement of estimated deficits.
3. Provision of ongoing maintenance requirements.

Where the dominant clinical problem relates to an inadequate circulating blood volume, the chief goal is to restore the circulation by supplying fluid that will be held preferentially in the circulating compartment of the ECF, that is, the plasma.

Three basic types of replacement fluid are available for clinical use:

- Electrolyte-free sugar solutions (e.g. 5% D-glucose in water).
- Isotonic solutions of sodium salts (e.g. 0.9% sodium chloride, which is 150 mM NaCl or normal saline).
- Isotonic salt solutions including colloid macromolecules (e.g. stable plasma protein solution).

The effectiveness of each of these solutions in restoring circulating volume can be deduced by reference to Fig. 2.3. Using first principles, considering 1 litre of each solution infused into a vein, the approximate distribution of volume would be as follows:

- The 5% dextrose solution would distribute approximately as does total body water, given that glucose is taken up freely by most cellular tissues. This would result in minimal expansion of the circulating blood volume, since the entire plasma and red cell volume is only about 12.5% of the total body water.
- A litre of normal saline would remain largely confined to the ECF, but of this only some 20% would remain in the plasma, the rest moving into the interstitial fluid compartment.
- A litre of protein-containing solution would be largely retained in the plasma compartment, since the oncotic effect of the colloid molecule would

serve to hold the added fluid inside the capillary endothelial barrier.

The urgency of fluid replacement and the choice of fluid used depends very much on the clinical circumstances, including the rate of development and nature of the deficit, assessed by clinical and biochemical parameters. Many cases of mild or chronic fluid and electrolyte deficiency can be corrected by simple measures, involving cessation of the causative disturbance, and oral replacement of fluid and electrolytes found to be deficient. In more acute or severe situations, intravenous therapy will be necessary. In either case, attention needs also to be given to prevent recurrence of the initiating disturbance.

Body fluids and nephron function box 4

Treatment

The clinicians caring for Joanne considered that her circulation was significantly affected by her prolonged diuretic use, and that a period of intravenous therapy would be the most effective way of restoring her circulation. She was admitted to hospital and the diuretics were ceased. She was given 1 litre of normal saline intravenously every 12 h for 48 h, with 30 mmol potassium chloride added to each litre.

Her symptoms rapidly resolved, and her plasma biochemistry normalized. She received counselling about the importance of refraining from further use of diuretic medications, and was given support and advice about her perceived weight and swelling problems. Her family doctor was involved in following her up in these matters.

Self-assessment case study

A 43-year-old woman is referred to the electrolyte clinic for further evaluation. She recently saw her family doctor complaining of weakness and tiredness, and a routine biochemical check revealed a low plasma potassium (*2.6 mmol/L). She has been generally well in the past, though always prone to light-headedness, especially in hot weather. She has recently experienced weakness on sustained use of her upper limbs, such as when hanging out the washing. She takes no regular medications, and denies irregularities of bowel function.

Her physical examination shows a tired looking woman with mild weakness affecting especially the proximal muscles of the arms and legs. The mouth appears rather dry, though the skin is unremarkable. Jugular venous pressure is not visible with the patient reclining at 45°. The blood pressure is 105/70 lying and 90/65 standing and pulse rate is 100 beats/min in both positions.

At the time she is seen in the referral clinic, she is accompanied by the following biochemical profile:

*Sodium 131 mmol/L
*Potassium 2.6 mmol/L
*Chloride 96 mmol/L
*Bicarbonate 33 mmol/L
*Urea 9.2 mmol/L
Creatinine 0.11 mmol/L.

Urine electrolytes ('spot' sample):
Sodium 48 mmol/L
Potassium 26 mmol/L.

(*Values outside the normal range; see Appendix.)

After studying this chapter you should be able to answer the following questions.

① What features of the history and examination are suggestive of hypovolaemia?

② Although no drugs have been formally prescribed, what medication might the patient be taking of her own accord?

③ What biochemical analysis would help distinguish between furosemide (frusemide) and thiazide use?

④ How would surreptitious diuretic use best be excluded?

⑤ In this patient, the urine calcium excretion was found to be very low, and no drugs were detected in the urine. In which segment of the nephron would you predict that there was an inherited or acquired functional defect?

Answers see page 145

① List three features on physical examination suggestive of hypervolaemia (volume expansion).

② Indicate the expected change from normal in each of the following parameters during hypervolaemia: plasma renin, plasma aldosterone, plasma atrial natriuretic peptide, glomerular filtration rate.

③ What changes would you expect in the plasma potassium concentration and urinary excretion of potassium during prolonged treatment with high dose spironolactone?

④ A 500-mL transfusion of whole blood is given to a patient with shock. The transfused blood has a haematocrit (packed cell volume) of 42%. Immediately after transfusion, what is the change in total intracellular fluid volume and extracellular fluid volume in the patient?

Answers see page 145

WATER BALANCE AND REGULATION OF OSMOLALITY

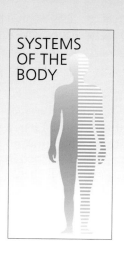

SYSTEMS
OF THE
BODY

Chapter objectives

After studying this chapter you should be able to:

① Define the normal range for plasma osmolality.

② Outline the mechanisms by which the kidney can concentrate the urine (during underhydration) and dilute the urine (during overhydration).

③ Explain the feedback mechanisms for the control of plasma osmolality, and the role of vasopressin (antidiuretic hormone).

④ Outline the differential diagnosis of polyuria, and explain some mechanisms involved in conditions associated with impaired capacity to concentrate the urine.

⑤ Give a differential diagnosis of hypernatraemia.

⑥ Describe the mechanisms involved in conditions involving impaired ability to dilute the urine.

⑦ Give a differential diagnosis of hyponatraemia.

3

Introduction

The previous chapter was largely concerned with the mechanisms whereby the kidney regulates body sodium balance. The point was made that the volume of the extracellular fluid (ECF) is largely determined by body sodium content, and hence adjustments to the renal sodium excretion rate have a major bearing on the ECF volume. We explained that, for the most part, alterations in tubular sodium transport are accompanied by parallel movements of water (though not necessarily in the same tubular segment) such that no net change in body fluid osmolality generally results from these adjustments.

In this chapter, we consider the mechanisms whereby water is handled by the kidney, independent of movements of sodium. These principles will give rise to an understanding of how the kidney is able to concentrate the urine by retaining water, or dilute the urine by excreting water as circumstances demand. It will also lead to an understanding of the origin of the clinical problems of polyuria, hypernatraemia and hyponatraemia.

See box 1.

Causes and assessment of polyuria

In principle, a high urine flow rate may be produced either by a primary increase in solute excretion or by a primary increase in water excretion.

Polyuria caused by solute diuresis results from the delivery of a high load of solute through the nephron, either as a result of filtration of a poorly reabsorbed solute, or of blunted reabsorption of a solute normally transported out of the tubular fluid. (Note that increased glomerular filtration rate (GFR) *per se* is not a common cause of polyuria, largely because of glomerulotubular balance; see Chapter 2). The first mechanism applies to the osmotic diuresis produced by infusions of mannitol, which cannot be reabsorbed from the nephron and hence traps water osmotically within the tubular lumen, resulting in a high urine flow rate. Osmotic diuresis can also occur during disease states, notably in uncontrolled diabetes mellitus. In this case, increased plasma glucose concentrations result in the filtration of a glucose load greater than that which can be reabsorbed by the proximal tubule glucose reabsorption mechanism (saturation of the sodium–glucose cotransport carrier), leading to **glycosuria** accompanied by increased water flow because of the osmotic effect of the glucose trapped in the lumen. This mechanism accounts for the polyuria and dehydration encountered in newly presenting or uncontrolled insulin-dependent diabetes. A broadly

Water balance and regulation of osmolality box 1

A case of polyuria

Robert Underwood is a 46-year-old man who presents to a doctor in a suburban medical centre complaining of passing large volumes of urine which is virtually colourless ('like water'), accompanied by excessive thirst. He claims to be drinking 5 or more litres of water per day, and passing similar volumes of urine. These symptoms have been troubling him for several weeks. He denies a history of similar complaints in the past, and has never been diagnosed with diabetes. He has never had known kidney disease and states that his general health has been good, although he has had some 'emotional problems' over the years. The family history is unremarkable. He says he is a reformed smoker, and does not drink alcohol at all.

On examination he seems a little agitated but otherwise looks quite well. The skin, lips and mouth appear rather dry, but the blood pressure is normal at 130/80, the pulse 84 beats/min. The rest of the examination is normal. A urine specimen is obtained, which is a very pale colour, and on urinalysis proves to be negative for glucose, blood and protein. This specimen, as well as a sample of blood, is sent to the pathology laboratory.

The questions that arise in considering this case are:

① What might be causing his polyuria and thirst?

② What determines how concentrated the urine is under normal conditions?

similar mechanism is occasionally seen during the development of chronic renal failure, where high levels of urea have a diuretic effect.

The second mechanism for solute diuresis is that produced by the commonly used diuretic drugs, which act to block the specific mechanisms for sodium reabsorption in discrete segments of the nephron (see Chapter 2). Polyuria of this cause is most prominent soon after commencement of the diuretic drug.

Water-based or dilute polyuria has a quite different mechanism, and can arise in one of two ways. First, a high intake of water will lead directly to a high output of dilute urine, through mechanisms to be described in this chapter. While a history of excessive water drinking might be expected in this situation, covert overdrinking is sometimes encountered in patients with psychiatric disturbances (psychogenic polydipsia). An alternative mechanism for polyuria associated with

Table 3.1
Diagnostic approach to polyuria

Type	Examples	Plasma	Urine
Solute	Uncontrolled diabetes mellitus (solute, glucose)	Increased osmolality, hyperglycaemia	High osmolality, glycosuria
	Furosemide (frusemide) therapy (solute, NaCl)	Normal osmolality*	Variable osmolality, high Na
Water	Psychogenic polydipsia	Low–normal osmolality	Low osmolality
	Impaired urine concentration (central or nephrogenic DI)	High–normal osmolality	Low osmolality

*The plasma osmolality and sodium concentration may be normal, low or high during loop diuretic therapy, depending on the water intake. DI, diabetes insipidus.

dilute urine is when the primary disorder involves the kidney's inability to concentrate the urine normally. The physiological defects giving rise to this condition, known as diabetes insipidus, will be detailed further below.

Table 3.1 illustrates some differential features in the diagnostic approach to polyuria. Of particular interest in this case and for the subject matter of this chapter, is the differentiation between the two forms of water diuresis. While in both forms the urine is dilute with low osmolality, in the case where the diuresis is being driven by high water intake the plasma would be expected to have a low osmolality, resulting directly from excessive water reabsorption from the gut. In the case of impaired urinary concentration mechanisms, the plasma osmolality would be high since the primary problem is excessive loss of water from the ECF into the urine.

See box 2.

By reference to Table 3.1, Mr Underwood's polyuria cannot be attributed to glucose or sodium as solutes, but is a water diuresis. Since the plasma sodium and osmolality are above the normal range, we can deduce that his problem arises from impaired urine concentration mechanisms rather than forced water drinking.

Renal mechanisms for urine concentration

It is obvious that there is a wide range in the normal intake of water, and also in the normal loss of water through the lungs, skin and gut (these three being sources of 'insensible' water loss). Yet despite this, under normal circumstances the osmolality of the plasma is tightly regulated around a mean of 290 mosm/kg, the normal range being within 5 mosm/kg either way. The homeostatic maintenance of this set point for plasma osmolality implies that the kidney is capable of adjusting the rate of water excretion over a wide range, by generating a dilute urine when water is abundant or by generating a concentrated urine

Water balance and regulation of osmolality box 2

Biochemistry results

The results of Mr Underwood's biochemistry become available the following day. These are shown below:

*Sodium 154 mmol/L
Potasssium 4.2 mmol/L
*Chloride 114 mmol/L
Bicarbonate 30 mmol/L
*Urea 11.5 mmol/L
*Creatinine 0.13 mmol/L
Glucose 4.5 mmol/L
*Osmolality 312 mosm/kg.

Urine biochemistry
Sodium 26 mmol/L
Glucose 0 mmol/L
Osmolality 80 mosm/kg.

The questions now are:

① What pattern of polyuria is suggested by these results?

② What further history or investigations are appropriate?

(*Results outside the normal range; see Appendix.)

when water is scarce. As illustrated in Fig. 3.1, this corresponds in the first case to excretion of urine with an osmolality below 300 (50 mosm/kg being the most dilute urine possible), or in the second case to the production of urine with maximum water extracted (resulting in a typical maximum osmolality around 1200–1400 mosm/kg). We will first look at how the process of concentration is achieved.

In overview, there are two broad requirements for the kidney to be able to produce a urine more concentrated than the plasma (Fig. 3.2). First, a zone must be

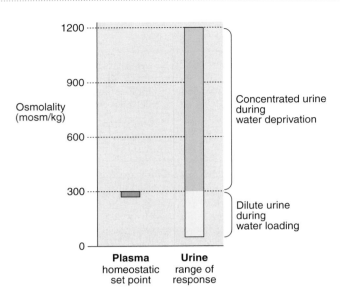

Fig. 3.1
Range of osmolality in plasma and urine.

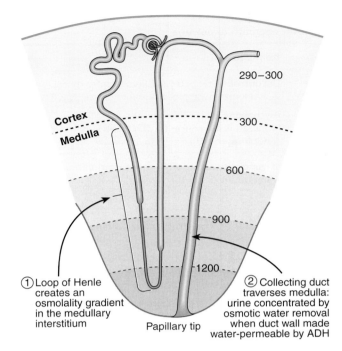

Fig. 3.2
Basic components of the urinary concentrating mechanism. Figures show osmolality of the tissue fluid (in mosm/kg) in different zones of the kidney. The loop of Henle sets up the tissue fluid osmolality gradient within the renal medulla, and the collecting duct traverses this gradient.

created within the renal medulla where the tissue fluid osmolality is high; second, the tubules forming the final segment of the nephron must conduct the urine through this concentrated zone, where water reabsorption can occur passively by osmosis (given that these segments can be made permeable to water). The first of these requirements is achieved by the operation of the loop of Henle as it dips into the renal medulla, while the second requirement is fulfilled by the collecting ducts as they pass from the cortex through the medulla on their way to deliver final urine to the renal pelvis. The mechanism whereby the water permeability of the collecting ducts can be increased where appropriate is through the action of circulating vasopressin (antidiuretic hormone; ADH).

Countercurrent multiplication by the loop of Henle

The principle whereby a loop structure can generate a longitudinal gradient of concentration (from the top ends of the loop to its bend) is illustrated in Fig. 3.3. Here the descending and ascending limbs of the loop are shown to be parallel and adjacent, with an intervening layer of tissue fluid lying between them. Flow in the two limbs is said to be countercurrent, in that fluid entering the descending limb (from the end of the proximal tubule) flows downward, while the flow in the adjacent ascending limb is upward, being delivered at the top into the early distal tubule. A second property of the model is that the walls of the descending limb are permeable to water, while those of the

ascending limb are impermeable to water. The third and key property of the system is that the walls of the ascending limb contain a pump mechanism capable of removing sodium chloride from the lumen and adding it to the surrounding interstitial fluid such that a gradient of 200 mosm/kg can be created across the tubular wall at any point. For clarity, the final effect of operating such a system in steady state is built up as a series of discontinuous steps in the diagram.

The flow step shows the effect of introducing some fluid from the proximal tubule into the descending limb (shown with an osmolality of 300 mosm/kg for convenience), and the effect this would have of displacing fluid in the loop in each stage of the model. The second step shows the effect of activating the pump in the ascending limb, creating the 200 mosm/kg gradient across its wall. The third step shows the effect of water movement by osmosis out of the descending limb such that the fluid in that limb attains the same osmolality as the tissue fluid surrounding the ascending limb. It can be seen that the sequential effect of admitting more fluid into the descending limb, and then activating the pump once more, is to multiply the effectiveness of the thick

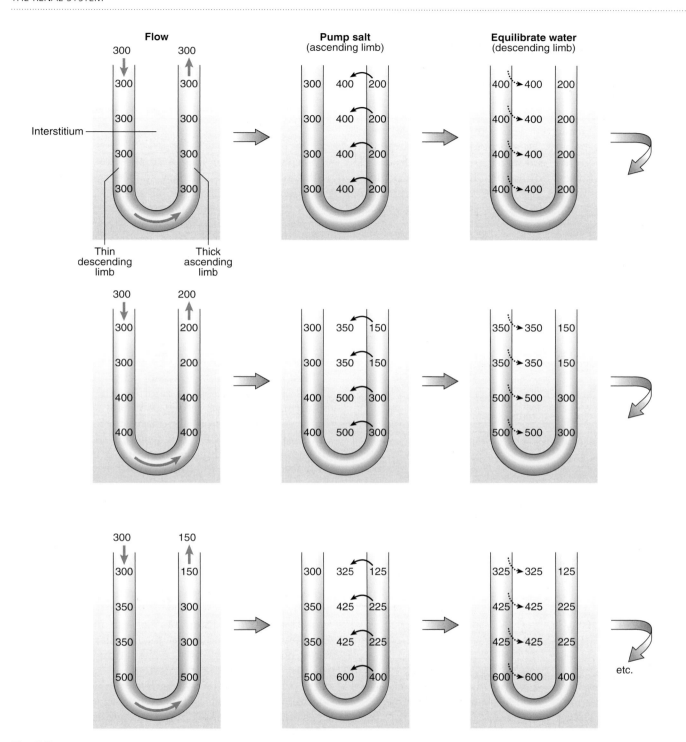

Fig. 3.3
Discontinuous model for the operation of the loop of Henle as a countercurrent multiplier. Figures are osmolality (mosm/kg). See text for detailed description.

ascending limb's pump mechanism in creating an area of high osmolality around the turn of the loop. In reality, the system operates continuously, resulting in the steady state situation shown in Fig. 3.4.

There are three important consequences of operation of this system. First, the fluid leaving the ascending limb of the loop ends up being quite hypo-osmolar (100 mosm/kg) compared to the fluid entering it.

Second, the osmolality near the bend of the loop is raised several fold above the osmolality of the entering fluid. Third, there is ultimately a continuous gradient of tissue osmolality from the 300 mosm/kg pervading near the top of the loop (in the renal cortex) to the 1200 mosm/kg achieved around the turn of the loop of Henle (though not all of this is due to salt accumulation; see below). This provides the environment through which the collecting ducts pass from the cortex through the medulla, providing an opportunity for water extraction from the collecting ducts by osmosis, given that their water permeability is sufficiently high.

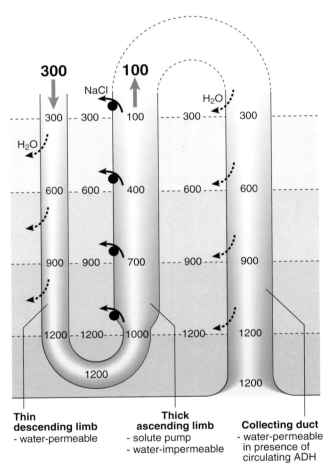

Fig. 3.4
Key properties and final outcome of loop of Henle function. The collecting duct properties are those during water deprivation when maximal urine concentration is being achieved. Figures are osmolality (mosm/kg). Note that in the thin descending limb and the collecting duct there is actually a small (5–10 mosm/kg) osmolality gradient between the lumen and the adjacent interstitium (which is higher) to make water move as shown.

From the above model, it can be deduced that three factors would increase the concentrating power achieved by the operation of the loop, namely:

- An increased length of the loop.
- An increased capacity of the pump in the thick ascending limb.
- A reduced flow rate through the loop.

Variations in the length of the loop underlie the differences in the urinary concentrating capacity between different mammalian species, related to the water availability in the habitat to which they are adapted. Variations in the power of the pump are seen clinically during the action of loop diuretics, such as furosemide (frusemide), which act to inhibit the thick ascending limb's solute reabsorptive capacity. Increases in flow through the loop are seen in volume-expanded states, during which concentrating capacity is reduced.

A number of refinements need to be added to the model to describe the actual situation in the mammalian kidney more fully.

First, the osmolality gradient within the medulla is not solely comprised of sodium chloride. Indeed, about half of the interstitial osmolality is contributed by urea. This relatively abundant small organic solute is 'trapped' within the renal medulla because of the different permeability of segments of the nephron to urea (being high in the thin descending and ascending limbs of the loop deep within the medulla, and in the medullary segment of the collecting duct when ADH is present, but low in the thick ascending limb and cortical distal tubule). Thus, under antidiuretic conditions, urea recycles from the medullary collecting duct (out) to the turn of the deep loops of Henle (in), adding to the inner medullary osmolality.

Second, it is clear that a capillary blood supply which crossed the kidney from cortex to medulla would allow for dissipation of the built up solute gradient by diffusion into the capillary blood. This does not occur because of the arrangement of the medullary capillaries themselves in loops, the vasa recta, which parallel the configuration for the juxtamedullary nephrons. Thus, while medullary solute does enter these vessels in the descending limb, it exits the capillaries in the ascending limb, while water moves in the opposite direction in each case (countercurrent exchange). Since, however, in the steady state the operation of the loop of Henle results in the loss of more solute than water from the tubular lumen, it follows that the vasa recta must remove more solute than water during their passage through the medulla.

A third refinement of the model is that it can be shown that countercurrent multiplication occurs even in the deepest hairpin part of the loop within the inner medulla, before the start of the thick ascending limb. The mechanisms involved here relate to the high water but low sodium permeabilities of the thin descending limb, and the reverse permeabilities of the thin ascending limb.

Action of ADH in the collecting ducts

The second component of the overall process involved in concentrating the urine is the action of ADH, also known as vasopressin. This peptide, which is released from the posterior part of the pituitary gland during conditions of water deprivation, acts to increase the water permeability of all segments of the collecting duct, from its earliest parts within the cortex (including the initial segments formed from the late distal tubules) through to the medullary segment as it traverses the outer and inner medulla on the way to emptying at the renal papilla. Thus, when ADH is present in the circulation, water is extensively reabsorbed from the collecting ducts in both the cortex and the medulla. Within the cortex, the maximum osmolality that can be achieved in the luminal fluid corresponds to the 300 mosm/kg present in the interstitial fluid in the cortex. Within the medulla, however, further water abstraction occurs until the osmolality of the urine in the terminal parts of the inner medullary collecting duct can reach the maximum osmolality achieved by the countercurrent mechanism at the tip of the renal papilla, namely about 1200 mosm/kg in man. This reabsorbed water is carried away by the capillaries forming the vasa recta, thus leaving the medullary interstitial osmolality gradient intact.

During states of overhydration, when ADH levels are low (see below), the urine remains dilute, since fluid emerging from the ascending limb of the loop is already hypotonic (see Fig. 3.4). It can be rendered somewhat more dilute by further removal of sodium chloride during passage through the distal tubules and collecting ducts which, under these conditions, are relatively impermeable to water. Hence the urinary osmolality can be lowered from the 100 mosm/kg emerging from the loop to as low as 50 mosm/kg under maximum water diuresis. (In fact, considerable water recovery does occur from the medullary collecting ducts during water diuresis since, although the water permeability is relatively low, the osmolality gradient favouring water reabsorption is high.)

In summary, Table 3.2 shows in simple form the factors required to achieve concentration of the urine on the one hand, and dilution of the urine on the other. The implications of interfering with these factors for the development of disturbed water balance during clinical conditions is discussed later in this chapter. For

Table 3.2
Conditions required for urinary concentration and dilution

To concentrate the urine
  Adequate solute delivery to the loop of Henle
  Normal function of the loop of Henle
  ADH release into the circulation
  ADH action on the collecting ducts

To dilute the urine
  Adequate solute delivery into the loop of Henle and early
    distal tubule
  Normal function of the loop of Henle and early distal tubule
  No ADH in the circulation

the moment it might be noted that loop diuretics clearly have the capacity to impair the kidney's ability to both concentrate and dilute the urine, while the thiazide diuretics, affecting only the component of urinary dilution which occurs in the early distal tubule within the cortex, interfere with maximum dilution of the urine but not with the mechanism for urinary concentration.

Feedback control of plasma osmolality

During conditions of water deprivation, plasma osmolality tends to rise. This osmolality change is detected by specialized neural cells in the hypothalamus called osmoreceptors which, on shrinking, convey electrical signals to adjacent hypothalamic structures, with two parallel outcomes. First, sensation of thirst is stimulated, leading the individual to seek and ingest water actively. Second, cells within the supraoptic and paraventricular hypothalamic nuclei are activated to synthesize ADH, which is transferred bound to a carrier protein neurophysin down specialized axons terminating in the posterior pituitary gland where it is released into the capillary blood. The ADH added to the circulation in this way reaches the kidney, where it acts to increase the water permeability of the collecting duct epithelial cells, resulting in enhanced water reabsorption from the tubular fluid. This, combined with greater intake of water stimulated by thirst, serves to bring the plasma osmolality down towards normal, whereupon osmoreceptor activity reduces and the water-retaining mechanisms are deactivated (Fig. 3.5).

The reverse sequence of events occurs after ingestion of a large volume of water. The plasma is initially diluted slightly as the water is reabsorbed from the gut. This results in a fall in osmolality which leads the osmoreceptor cells to reduce their activity, following which thirst is suppressed and ADH release is inhibited. These two measures lead to production by the kidney of a dilute urine of high volume, as tubular

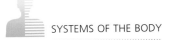
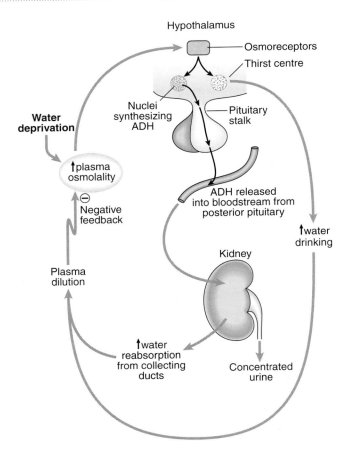

Fig. 3.5
Feedback control of plasma osmolality.

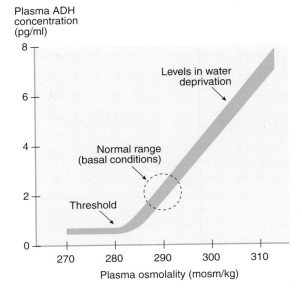

Fig. 3.6
Relationship between plasma osmolality and plasma concentration of ADH.

fluid diluted within the loop of Henle becomes further diluted as it passes through distal nephron segments, which remain impermeable to water in the absence of ADH. As the water load is rapidly excreted, plasma osmolality returns toward normal and baseline conditions are restored.

Figure 3.6 shows the relationship between the plasma osmolality and the concentration of ADH released into the plasma. It can be seen that the threshold for release of ADH is around 280 mosm/kg, only slightly below the normal set point for plasma osmolality (290 ± 5 mosm/kg). A steep linear rise in circulating ADH results as osmolality passes above 290, while ADH release is virtually zero below 280 mosm/kg.

Two factors make the ADH system very effective in the short-term regulation of plasma osmolality. First, ADH is a small peptide (nine amino acids) which has a very short half-life in the circulation, so that its action is not unduly prolonged following its release. Second, the release of ADH from the hypothalamus in response to osmoreceptor signals and its action within the kidney are extremely rapid events, such that the

system tracks minute-to-minute changes in the osmolality of the plasma, correcting them towards the norm without undue delays.

A variety of non-osmotic stimuli may also cause secretion of ADH, independent of the plasma osmolality. Thus, haemodynamic changes associated with a fall in circulating plasma volume are potent triggers for ADH release. These disturbances are signalled to the brainstem via the volume and pressure sensors located in the central circulation (see Chapter 2), and the result is an independent input into the ADH secretory cells in the hypothalamus, resulting as before in ADH release into the circulation. While stimuli such as hypovolaemia and hypotension can lead to very high levels of ADH in the plasma, the sensitivity of the system to these changes is less than to alterations in plasma osmolality. Thus, while a 1% rise in plasma osmolality is sufficient to trigger a rise in ADH secretion, a 5–10% decrease in blood volume or blood pressure is required to provoke its secretion. Changes of this order do occur, however, in states of circulatory collapse. In addition, other non-osmotic stimuli such as pain, nausea and stress may also provoke ADH release, while alcohol inhibits it.

Mechanism of ADH action in the kidney

Figure 3.7 shows the cellular events involved in the action of ADH in increasing the water permeability of the collecting duct. The ADH in the circulation binds to a specific receptor, named the V2 receptor which is

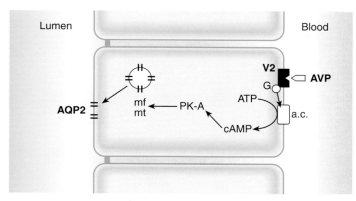

Fig. 3.7
Cellular mechanism of action of ADH in the collecting duct. AVP, arginine vasopressin (ADH); V2, vasopressin 2 receptor; G, G protein; a.c., adenyl cyclase; PK-A, protein kinase-A; mf, microfilaments; mt, microtubules; AQP2, aquaporin 2.

Table 3.3
Failure of urinary concentration

Mechanism	Clinical example
Failure to generate medullary concentration gradient:	
Poor solute delivery to the loop of Henle	Low GFR (chronic renal failure)
Impaired action of thick ascending limb of loop	Loop diuretic therapy (furosemide; frusemide)
Failure of ADH effect:	
No ADH released	Central DI (hypothalamic/ pituitary lesion)
No ADH action in kidney	Nephrogenic DI (collecting duct cell dysfunction)

DI, diabetes insipidus; GFR, glomerular filtration rate.

located on the basolateral membrane of the collecting duct epithelial cells. Through an intermediary G protein, this results in the activation of the membrane-bound enzyme adenyl cyclase, which catalyses the conversion of cellular ATP to cyclic AMP. This second messenger is responsible for activating protein kinases within the cytoplasm, which leads to the phosphorylation of certain proteins involved in the activity of cytoskeletal elements (myofilaments and myofibrils) located in the apical cell cytoplasm. These appear to mobilize vesicles lying below the apical cell membrane which contain preformed water channels comprising the specific channel protein aquaporin 2 (AQP2). Movement of these vesicles into the apical cell membrane results in the addition of AQP2 channels into that membrane, greatly increasing its water permeability. The relatively dilute tubular fluid is now able to move down an osmotic gradient through the cell cytoplasm and into the interstitial fluid and plasma across the basolateral membrane (the water permeability of which is due to the presence of aquaporins 3 and 4).

Two other intrarenal actions of ADH have been defined, both of which amplify its capacity to cause concentration of the urine. First, there is evidence that ADH can increase the activity of the sodium chloride reabsorptive mechanism located in the thick ascending limb of the loop of Henle; and second, ADH increases the permeability of the inner medullary collecting duct to urea. Both of these actions lead to an intensification of the medullary interstitial concentration gradient.

Finally, it is important to mention here that ADH has a separate action, mediated by a different receptor (the V1 receptor, involving intracellular calcium mobiliza-

tion), by which it promotes vasoconstriction of arterioles throughout the body. This vasoconstrictor action of the hormone increases the blood pressure in the central circulation at the same time as its renal tubular actions serve to retain water. Both actions therefore counteract the circulatory collapse associated with hypovolaemia or dehydration.

Failure to concentrate the urine

We can return now to an analysis of Robert Underwood's apparent failure of urine concentrating capacity. It follows from the above discussion that failure of the normal urine concentrating mechanism may result from any of the causes listed in Table 3.3. It is usually quite straightforward to exclude the first causes, involving either established renal failure or the presence of loop diuretics, either of which can lead to inadequate generation of the medullary concentration gradient by the loop of Henle. It is less easy, however, to distinguish whether impaired concentration results from failure to manufacture or release ADH from the brain (hypothalamic or central diabetes insipidus), or from failure of ADH to act appropriately on the renal collecting duct cells (nephrogenic diabetes insipidus).

Both indirect and direct methods for distinguishing between these two conditions are available. First, as shown in Fig. 3.8, a water deprivation test can be performed. In this test, the subject is initially well hydrated such that the urine osmolality is quite low. Urine osmolality is monitored as the patient is observed closely during a period of water deprivation. While the normal subject will develop increased urine osmolality after some 9–12 h of water deprivation as a result of endogenous ADH release, in neither form of diabetes insipidus (DI) will substantial urine concen-

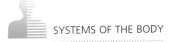

WATER BALANCE AND REGULATION OF OSMOLALITY

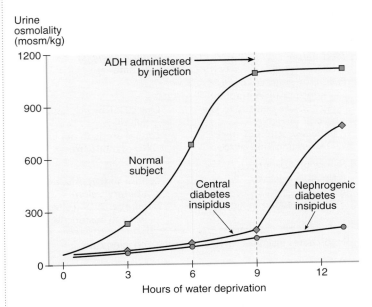

Fig. 3.8
Urinary omolality *versus* time during a water deprivation test. Characteristic patterns are shown for a normal subject, and for patients with central and nephrogenic diabetes insipidus.

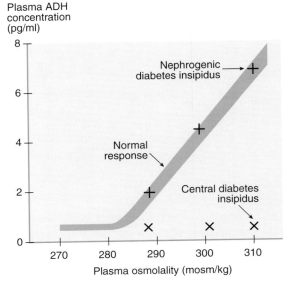

Fig. 3.9
Position of patients with central and nephrogenic diabetes insipidus on the plasma ADH *versus* plasma osmolality graph.

tration occur. Administration of an exogenous dose of ADH at this point will produce a urine concentrating response in the patient with central DI, where there is lack of hypothalamic hormone synthesis, while the patient with nephrogenic DI will have negligible response, reflecting impaired collecting duct capacity to respond to the hormone. Figure 3.9 shows where these two classes of patients would appear on the plasma osmolality *versus* plasma ADH concentration graph. As the plasma osmolality rises, the patient with central DI is unable to raise the near-zero levels of ADH in the plasma appreciably, while the ADH concentration rise in nephrogenic DI may be within the normal range.

The causes of central DI include tumours, trauma, irradiation or cerebrovascular accidents which destroy the relevant regions of the hypothalamus or the pituitary stalk or the posterior pituitary itself. Inflammatory conditions such as sarcoidosis can occasionally produce the same effect. Causes of nephrogenic DI, on the other hand, include either inherited or acquired problems with the collecting duct ADH response mechanism shown in Fig. 3.7. Inherited conditions have been defined in which there is faulty structure and impaired function of either the V2 receptor protein on the basolateral membrane, or of AQP2 water channels in the apical membrane. Acquired forms of nephrogenic DI can occur when the collecting duct system is affected by infection or obstruction, or where

there is interference with the intracellular steps after generation of cyclic AMP, preventing aquaporin translocation into the apical membrane. Examples of this latter mechanism include nephrogenic DI during hypokalaemia, hypercalcaemia and lithium therapy.
See box 3.

Differential diagnosis of hypernatraemia

A useful generalization is that disturbances in ECF sodium *concentration* reflect primary alterations in body water content. In contrast, as discussed in Chapter 2, primary disturbances in body sodium *content* are usually accompanied by parallel changes in the ECF volume status, detected by clinical examination rather than plasma analysis.

When the plasma sodium concentration (and hence osmolality) are increased above normal levels, there is usually a total body water deficit. While this can arise occasionally through inadequate water intake alone, the cause is usually excessive loss of water from the body. As shown in Table 3.4, in some settings this water loss is accompanied by a degree of salt loss, although the water loss in these cases is disproportionately greater. This may occur through the kidney, as for example during diuresis induced by osmotic agents or loop-acting drugs (in water-restricted patients), through the skin (during excessive sweating), or via the gut (during colonic diarrhoea, especially in children).

Water balance and regulation of osmolality box 3

The diagnosis

Mr Underwood's history, physical examination and biochemical results were reviewed, looking for clues to one of the known mechanisms for impaired urinary concentration. Severe renal impairment was excluded by the virtually normal plasma creatinine concentration, and loop diuretics had never been prescribed or taken by the patient.

Initially, investigations were directed towards excluding the possibility of hypothalamic DI by arranging for an assay of plasma ADH level at a time when the patient was dehydrated and hyper-osmolar, as at presentation. A cerebral CT scan was also organized, looking for evidence of structural damage in the area of the hypothalamus or pituitary fossa.

At this point, however, the patient volunteered that he had been receiving psychiatric treatment for 1 month, following his presentation in an agitated and hypomanic state. He had started on lithium car-bonate tablets, 500 mg bd, and therapy was currently being stabilized in conjunction with his psychiatrist. Indeed, a plasma lithium concentration of 0.9 mmol/l had recently been obtained by his psychiatrist, with whom contact was now made.

A diagnosis of lithium-induced nephrogenic DI was therefore made. Consistent with this, the plasma ADH concentration result later came back in the high normal range, appropriate for the elevated plasma osmolality. The cerebral CT scan proved to be normal.

In this situation, management consists of several steps: the patient was advised always to maintain an adequate water intake, but not to drink more than thirst demanded. If indeed the psychiatric judgement was that lithium therapy should be continued, given its efficacy in controlling the mood swings of **bipolar affective disorder**, close monitoring of the resultant plasma lithium levels was recommended to maintain the serum lithium within and at the lower end of the recommended therapeutic range (0.4–0.8 mmol/L). Finally, if polyuria and thirst persisted and were troublesome to the patient, a trial of amiloride therapy could be considered. Experimental and clinical evidence suggests that this agent blocks uptake of lithium as well as sodium through the apical cation channel in the cortical collecting duct, mitigating the extent of lithium's interference with the intracellular steps in ADH.

Table 3.4
Differential diagnosis of hypernatraemia

Water deficit with proportionately smaller sodium deficit
  Renal: osmotic or loop diuretic (during water restriction)
  Extrarenal: skin (excessive sweating)
       gut (colonic diarrhoea)

Water deficit alone
  Renal: central or nephrogenic diabetes insipidus

Sodium loading with normal or reduced body water
  Enteral or parenteral alimentation
  Intravenous or oral salt administration

Note that in all cases there is usually some blunting of the normal thirst mechanism and/or restricted access to water.

Water loss unaccompanied by electrolyte depletion does occur in DI, where there is a failure of the normal operation of the ADH system. As described above, this may occur because of hypothalamic failure to synthesize ADH (central DI) or through renal tubular insensitivity to ADH present in the circulation (nephrogenic DI).

Less commonly, hypernatraemia can result from sodium loading, with either normal or reduced body water content. This is an unusual occurrence, and may occur during **enteral** or **parenteral alimentation** with hyperosmotic solutions, or during administration of dietary or therapeutic supplements containing high salt content.

Note that whatever the underlying cause, sustained or severe hypernatraemia must reflect an impaired thirst mechanism, such as that associated with brain damage or stroke, and/or impaired availability of, or access to, water. When thirst mechanisms and water availability are not limiting, the subject will normally drink sufficient water to keep the osmolality from rising very high.

It is clear from the above analysis that the finding of hypernatraemia itself gives no guide as to the total body sodium status. This must be independently assessed using clinical clues, including history and a physical examination seeking signs of hypovolaemia or hypervolaemia (see Chapter 2).

Failure to dilute the urine

The reverse scenario of that described in the previous sections of this chapter occurs when the ECF becomes hypo-osmolar because of impairment of the mechanisms normally involved in excreting excess ingested water; that is, in diluting the urine. As summarized in Table 3.2, this process requires adequate delivery of fil-trate through the segments of the nephron capable of

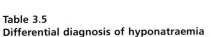

WATER BALANCE AND REGULATION OF OSMOLALITY

3

lowering the osmolality of the luminal fluid by removing sodium while remaining impermeable to water. These properties are possessed by the ascending limb of the loop of Henle and the early (convoluted) part of the distal tubule. Secondly, ADH secretion must be suppressed appropriately by the low plasma osmolality so that water is not reabsorbed from the collecting duct system.

In assessing the patient with inappropriate water retention, it is thus necessary first to rule out renal failure (low GFR); second, to exclude use of diuretic drugs acting on the thick ascending limb (e.g. furosemide; frusemide) or the early distal tubule (e.g. thiazides); and third, to determine that ADH is not being released into the circulation. In regard to the latter, it must be remembered that ADH release can be triggered not only by a rise in plasma osmolality, but also by non-osmotic stimuli such as hypovolaemia, hypotension, nausea, stress and pain. Sometimes these stimuli are present without elevation of the plasma osmolality, resulting in water retention sufficient to drive the plasma osmolality below the normal range.

Differential diagnosis of hyponatraemia

These considerations are most commonly brought to bear in assessing the clinical problem of hyponatraemia. Nearly all of the hyponatraemic states are associated with sustained action of ADH in retaining water from the collecting ducts, despite the presence of hypo-osmolality which would otherwise be expected to switch off ADH release. The main exception is forced water drinking, such as that which occurs in psychogenic polydipsia: in this situation the primary excess of ingested water, and slight expansion of ECF volume, both act to switch off ADH, such that maximal urine dilution occurs. Hyponatraemia only develops to the extent that water ingestion continues at a rate exceeding its maximal excretion rate through the kidney.

The other causes of hyponatraemia are summarized in Table 3.5. Relative water retention may occur in conditions where there is a sodium deficit and hypovolaemia. This is due most commonly to sodium losses through the gastrointestinal tract (e.g. vomiting) or via the kidney (e.g. during diuretic action). As previously mentioned, in the case of loop and early distal acting diuretics, sodium loss is compounded by interference with the mechanisms for generating dilute urine in these nephron segments. Deficiency of **adrenocortical hormones** also results in renal sodium wasting. In all of these conditions, ADH is activated through the mechanism of hypovolaemia consequent

Table 3.5
Differential diagnosis of hyponatraemia

Sodium deficit with relative water retention
Renal: thiazides and loop diuretics (during water drinking), adrenocortical failure
Extrarenal: gut (e.g. vomiting)

Water retention alone
SIADH: ectopic ADH secretion from tumour, lung disease, CNS disease, drugs
Hypothyroidism

Sodium retention with relatively greater water retention
Generalized oedema states: congestive cardiac failure, cirrhosis, nephrotic syndrome
Chronic renal failure

Note that psychogenic polydipsia and other forms of forced water drinking are excluded from this table. SIADH, syndrome of inappropriate ADH secretion.

upon ECF volume reduction. The stage is thus set for persistence of hyponatraemia until the sodium deficit is restored.

Water retention without a major change in body sodium can occur where ADH levels are elevated with neither an osmotic nor a hypovolaemic stimulus. In the syndrome of inappropriate ADH secretion (SIADH), ADH is released into the circulation either from an ectopic site, such as a hormone-secreting tumour (e.g. lung cancer), or from the posterior pituitary, secondary to non-malignant lung disease which may stimulate intrathoracic receptors so as to mimic volume depletion. A variety of drugs may also stimulate central ADH release, e.g. phenothiazines, vincristine, cyclophosphamide. In SIADH, there is hyponatraemia with plasma hypo-osmolality, but with a urine which remains inappropriately concentrated, i.e. not maximally dilute. The urine sodium concentration is relatively high, which excludes plasma volume contraction in which it would be low.

A final category of hyponatraemia is that which arises when there is salt retention, but relatively greater water retention. This can occur during any of the conditions causing systemic oedema, such as congestive cardiac failure, nephrotic syndrome and cirrhosis. The water retention in these cases is partly because of the impaired GFR and avid proximal sodium and water reabsorption, which limit delivery of solute through the diluting segments of the nephron, and partly because of ADH release into the circulation. ADH secretion in these conditions is triggered by a reduction in the 'effective' arterial blood volume related to the impaired haemodynamics prevailing in each condition (see also Chapter 6).

The management of hyponatraemia depends first on defining the aetiology and reversing the causative condition wherever possible. This being done, treatment for hypovolaemic states involves volume replacement with intravenous sodium chloride infusions. For hypervolaemic conditions, sodium restriction accompanied by even tighter water restriction is necessary. In SIADH and related conditions, restriction of water alone is the mainstay of treatment.

Again it is worth reiterating that a low plasma sodium concentration generally reflects the relative excess of water in the ECF, and gives no reliable guide to the total body sodium and volume status. This must be determined from the history and by physical examination, using guidelines provided in Chapter 2.

Self-assessment case study

A consultation is requested on a hospitalized patient because of hyponatraemia. The patient was admitted 72 h before following a motor vehicle accident in which injuries were sustained to the chest and head. There is no evidence of skull fracture, although two ribs are broken on the left chest wall. The patient has been rather drowsy and confused since admission, although there are no localizing neurological signs. He has received some intravenous fluids since admission and there is no clinical evidence of hypervolaemia or hypovolaemia.

The plasma sodium level has fallen from 139 mmol/L on admission to 124 mmol/L, with an osmolality on the second occasion of 256 mosm/kg. A single urine sample has been obtained, and this shows a sodium concentration of 54 mmol/L and an osmolality of 460 mosm/kg.

After studying this chapter you should be able to answer the following questions:

① Does this patient show inappropriate failure to concentrate the urine or inappropriate failure to dilute the urine?

② What laboratory evidence confirms the clinical impression that he is not hypovolaemic?

③ What influences might be acting to determine the plasma level of antidiuretic hormone (ADH) in this clinical setting?

④ What management would you suggest for the hyponatraemia in this context?

Answers see page 145

Self-assessment questions

① What properties of the loop of Henle are critical to its operation as a countercurrent multiplication system?

② What changes in which parameters of the loop of Henle function would be expected to decrease its capacity to generate a hypertonic medullary interstitium?

③ Name, in order, the physiological changes which occur after ingestion of a large volume of water leading to its excretion shortly afterwards through the kidney.

④ Name the sequence of cellular actions which follow binding of antidiuretic hormone (ADH) to its receptor in the collecting duct of the kidney.

Answers see page 146

ACID–BASE BALANCE AND REGULATION OF pH

SYSTEMS OF THE BODY

Chapter objectives

After studying this chapter you should be able to:

① Define the normal range for plasma pH.

② Explain the role of the kidney in the steady state elimination of acid produced daily by metabolism.

③ Outline the defence mechanisms which act to prevent an abrupt change in pH in response to an acid load.

④ Describe the mechanism for acid transport in the different nephron segments.

⑤ Recognize the clinical and biochemical features of metabolic acidosis, list some causes and give an approach to the differential diagnosis.

⑥ Recognize metabolic alkalosis, list some causes, and explain the pathophysiology of this disturbance during prolonged vomiting.

Introduction

Just as the kidney is a critical organ in defending the normal set points for extracellular fluid (ECF) volume, osmolality and potassium concentration, it also plays a central role in the homeostasis of the plasma pH. While chemical buffering mechanisms and respiratory elimination of carbon dioxide are important in immediate responses to disturbances in acid–base balance, it falls to the kidney to make long-term adjustments in the rate of acid excretion which allows the external balance with respect to hydrogen ion concentration to be maintained. This chapter will focus on the mechanisms whereby the kidney achieves this role, and the origin of some disturbances of this system in disease.

See box 1.

The clue in this case that there is a disturbance of acid–base metabolism is that the bicarbonate concentration, representing the base component of the principal physiological buffer system, is greatly reduced below the normal range. This is consistent with acid accumulation in the ECF, for which we must explore both the cause and the consequences.

The key parameter involved in acid–base regulation is the concentration of H^+ in the ECF. The physiological set point for this parameter is 40 nmol/L, usually expressed (using the negative base 10 logarithm) as the pH, which is normally 7.40. So important is homeostasis of this parameter to the normal operation of metabolism and cellular function that pH is tightly regulated in the range 7.38–7.42, although a somewhat wider range is compatible with life (7.0–7.8).

Two forms of acid are generated as a result of normal metabolic processes. Oxidative metabolism produces a large amount of CO_2 daily, and this so-called 'volatile acid' is excreted through the lungs. Carbon dioxide effectively acts as an acid in body fluids because of the following reactions:

$$CO_2 + H_2O \overset{c.a.}{\rightleftharpoons} H_2CO_3 \rightleftharpoons H^+ + HCO_3^-$$

The first reaction (formation of carbonic acid, H_2CO_3) is the rate-limiting step and is normally slow, but in the presence of the enzyme carbonic anhydrase (c.a.) the reaction is greatly accelerated. The subsequent ionization of carbonic acid proceeds almost instantaneously. This equation can be rearranged to enhance its physiological utility in the form shown in Fig. 4.1, as the Henderson–Hasselbalch equation.

The other form of acid, the so-called 'non-volatile acid', results from the metabolism of dietary protein, resulting in the accumulation of some 70 mmol of acid per day in an average adult on a typical western meat-containing diet.

Acid–base balance and regulation of pH box 1

A case of acidosis

Mrs Mary Loy is a 48-year-old woman of Chinese background who has been sent by her family doctor to the Emergency Department because of his concern about her clinical condition and some biochemical results.

She had been complaining for some weeks of increasing lethargy, an extensive rash and 'heavy breathing'. She had been receiving treatment for 4 years for systemic lupus erythematosus (SLE), a multiorgan autoimmune condition for which a consultant rheumatologist had prescribed prednisone. However, Mrs Loy confessed to having discontinued this medication some 10 months earlier because she was unhappy about its side effects.

On examination she was febrile, unwell and had an erythematous rash on her face and limbs. Her blood pressure was 110/80, pulse rate 100 beats/min and respiratory rate 20/min, the breathing being deep and sighing. The referring doctor's letter indicated that he had obtained a urinalysis result that morning showing: pH 7, blood +++ and protein ++.

He had also obtained plasma biochemistry the previous day, the results of which are as follows:

Sodium 135 mmol/L
*Potassium 3.1 mmol/L
*Chloride 113 mmol/L
*Bicarbonate 13 mmol/L
Urea 8.0 mmol/L
Creatinine 0.09 mmol/L.

The family doctor is particularly concerned about the low bicarbonate, which he interprets as a sign of acid build-up, and seeks full evaluation of her clinical and metabolic problem.

(*Results outside the normal range; see Appendix.)

The most important mechanism preventing change in the pH of the ECF is the carbonic acid/bicarbonate buffer system outlined above. The importance of this buffer pair relates to certain key properties: bicarbonate is present in a relatively high concentration in the ECF (24 mmol/L) and the components of the buffer system are effectively under physiological control: the CO_2 by the lungs, and the bicarbonate by the kidneys. These relationships are illustrated in Fig. 4.1.

It is clear from this relationship that a shift in pH can be brought about by either a primary change in the bicarbonate concentration (metabolic disturbances) or in the partial pressure of CO_2 in the blood (respiratory disturbances). However, it can also be seen that alterations in each of these parameters may represent a compensatory change whereby either the kidney or the lung can act to limit the extent of pH change which would occur because of a primary disturbance in respiratory function or in metabolism, respectively. The patterns of resulting clinical acid–base disturbances will be discussed later in this chapter.

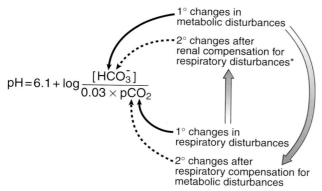

Fig. 4.1

Effect of changes in HCO_3^- and pCO_2 on net pH of the plasma. This is an applied version of the Henderson–Hasselbalch equation. Normal plasma $[HCO_3^-] = 24$ mmol/L, normal $pCO_2 = 40$ mmHg, giving a normal plasma pH of 7.40. The pH will return to 7.40 as long as the ratio of $[HCO_3^-] : [0.03 \times pCO_2]$ is $20 : 1$. *Note that changes in HCO_3^- concentration are also made as part of the renal correction of sustained metabolic acid–base disturbances as long as the kidney itself is not the cause of the primary disturbance.

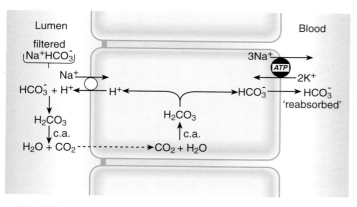

Fig. 4.2

Mechanism of proximal tubular bicarbonate reabsorption. Details of the bicarbonate exit mechanism across the basolateral membrane are not shown in this or subsequent figures. c.a., carbonic anhydrase.

Role of the kidney in H⁺ balance

Before we can make further progress in analysing the acid–base problem in our patient, it is necessary to consider the role the kidney plays in maintaining acid–base balance under normal conditions. Given that bicarbonate buffer is freely filtered at the glomerulus and that there is a daily load of non-volatile acid to be excreted into the urine, there must be two components to the nephron's task: reabsorption of filtered bicarbonate, and addition of net acid to the tubular fluid.

Bicarbonate reabsorption

Bicarbonate is the principal physiological buffer in the plasma and it is freely filtered at the glomerulus. If this bicarbonate were not fully reabsorbed by the tubular system, there would be ongoing losses of essential buffer into the urine, resulting in progressive acidification of the body fluids as metabolic acid production continued. In fact, bicarbonate excretion is essentially zero under normal conditions because of the extensive and efficient reabsorption of bicarbonate, principally in the proximal tubule as shown in Fig. 4.2.

As discussed in Chapter 2, the cells in this tubular segment contain a sodium–hydrogen exchange carrier molecule known as NHE-3 in the apical cell membrane. As sodium enters the cell from the luminal fluid down its electrochemical gradient via this carrier, it effectively removes hydrogen ions from the cell cytoplasm and adds them to the luminal fluid. The hydrogen ions are generated within the cell by the action of the enzyme carbonic anhydrase, which catalyses the reaction between CO_2 and water to produce carbonic acid. This rapidly breaks down to produce the hydrogen ions that are secreted into the lumen, and a bicarbonate ion which is transported across the basolateral cell membrane into the plasma. (Note that this is equivalent to saying that the dissociation of cellular water yields a hydrogen ion and a hydroxyl ion, which reacts with cytoplasmic CO_2 under the influence of carbonic anhydrase to produce the bicarbonate for basolateral extrusion.) Carbonic anhydrase also exists on the brush border membrane on the luminal surface of these cells. Here it catalyses the breakdown of carbonic acid formed as the secreted hydrogen ion reacts with filtered bicarbonate, releasing water and CO_2 which passes freely across the cell membrane, allowing the cycle to repeat.

The net outcome of this process is that the filtered sodium bicarbonate passing through the proximal tubule is effectively reabsorbed, although the bicarbonate added to the plasma in a given turn of the cycle is not the same one appearing in the lumen with sodium. This process accounts for reabsorption of some 85% of filtered bicarbonate, and operates at a high capacity but generates a low gradient of hydrogen ion concentration across the epithelium, with the luminal pH falling only slightly from 7.4 at the glomerulus to around 7.0 at the end of the proximal tubule. This is both because of the presence of carbonic anhydrase in the luminal compartment and because the epithelium is 'leaky' to hydrogen ions.

Net acid excretion

It is important to understand that the process described above has not done anything to remove net acid from the body, since the fate of the secreted H^+ in this segment is effectively to conserve most of the filtered bicarbonate. Under circumstances requiring removal of net acid from the body, the tubules must still carry out two more steps.

- Secrete further acid into the tubular lumen beyond that needed to reabsorb all filtered bicarbonate.
- Provide a buffer in the tubular fluid to assist in the removal of this acid (this is necessary since the maximum acidification which can be achieved in the lumen – around pH 4.5 – would not allow for excretion of the metabolic acid load needing elimination).

These two requirements are fulfilled in more distal nephron segments. As shown in Figs 4.3 and 4.4, acid is secreted into the lumen of the late distal tubule and collecting ducts by an H^+-ATPase located in the apical cell membrane. This pump has been found in the intercalated cells within the cortical collecting duct and in the apical membrane of the outer medullary collecting duct cells. The H^+ undergoing secretion in this way is generated within the tubular cells by a reaction facilitated by carbonic anhydrase, as described for the proximal tubule. Again, the bicarbonate generated within the cell by this process passes across the basolateral membrane (actually via a chloride–bicarbonate exchange carrier not shown in Fig. 4.3) into the plasma. However, here the bicarbonate does not replace a filtered bicarbonate molecule, but represents a 'new' bicarbonate, effectively counteracting the consumption of buffer which would have occurred had the excreted acid been retained in the body.

Two types of buffer are involved in excretion of this net acid. The glomerular filtrate contains a limited amount of non-bicarbonate buffer which is capable of taking up some of the H^+, as shown in Fig. 4.3. The main molecule involved is monohydrogen phosphate

(HPO_4^{2-}), which is titrated in the distal lumen to dihydrogen phosphate ($H_2PO_4^-$), which is excreted in the urine with sodium. This reaction has limited capacity (removing up to 30 mmol of H^+/day) and tends to proceed as the urine pH falls along the distal nephron segments, typically from 7 down to 6 and below, the

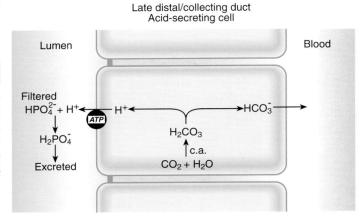

Fig. 4.3
Titration of filtered buffer (phosphate) by acid secreted in the distal nephron. Movements of filtered sodium ions are not shown. c.a., carbonic anhydrase.

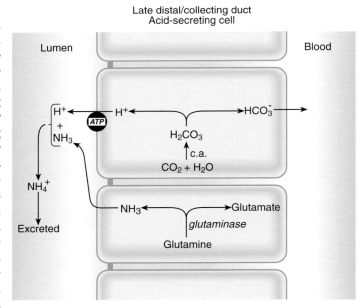

Fig. 4.4
Titration of manufactured buffer (ammonia) by acid secreted in the distal nephron. Ammonia synthesis is shown for convenience occurring in an adjacent distal cell; in fact, it is largely synthesized in proximal tubular cells. c.a., carbonic anhydrase.

pK (acid dissociation constant) of this buffer system being 6.8. This form of excreted H^+ is sometimes called 'titratable acid' as it can be quantitated by back-titrating a specimen of urine.

The other form of buffer involved in removal of secreted acid is that manufactured by the kidney itself, namely ammonia (NH_3). Renal tubular cells, especially those of the proximal tubule, contain the enzyme glutaminase, which catalyses the production of NH_3 from the nitrogen-rich amino acid glutamine. Ammonia itself is a lipid-soluble gas, which diffuses freely through the kidney tissue and is converted to its protonated form ammonium (NH_4^+) in acidic environments (it is also concentrated in the renal medulla by recirculation in the loop of Henle). As the luminal pH falls from the proximal to the distal nephron segments, the NH_4^+ becomes increasingly 'trapped' in the luminal fluid compartment where it is washed away into the urine, associated with chloride ions. Again this constitutes removal of an unwanted H^+ from the body, with restoration of a 'new' bicarbonate molecule to the ECF. The importance of this mechanism for acid excretion is that it is linked to an abundant and regulated source of buffer production (NH_3) of essentially unlimited capacity. Thus, under conditions of acid build-up (especially chronic acidosis), NH_3 synthesis is stimulated and acid excretion (as ammonium) is greatly increased, allowing systemic acid–base balance to be maintained.

Note that despite the action of NH_3 to buffer the build-up of free acid in the late segments of the nephron, the pH of the tubular fluid does fall along the collecting duct system, resulting in final urinary pH as low as 4.5. This occurs both because the distal nephron is relatively impermeable to H^+ and because there is no carbonic anhydrase in the luminal compartment in these tubular segments. This means that the dehydration of carbonic acid formed in the lumen is slow, allowing H^+ to accumulate.

In summary, under conditions of normal dietary protein consumption, a slightly alkaline plasma pH of 7.40 is maintained despite the generation of about 70 mmol of hydrogen ion (as non-volatile acid) per day. The kidney's role in maintaining this pH homeostasis is achieved by generating an acidic urine in which the net daily excess of acid can be removed. It does this in the following ways.

- Reabsorbing all bicarbonate buffer filtered into the urine.
- Secreting H^+ for excretion with filtered buffers such as phosphate.
- Secreting H^+ for excretion with the manufactured buffer ammonia.

Disturbances of acid–base balance: acidosis

Following from the above principles, we can now examine how the kidney is involved in the response to acid–base disturbances, and will consider first the situation of excess acid accumulation, or acidosis. This may arise as a result of either of two primary disturbances.

Respiratory acidosis

Respiratory acidosis results from the accumulation of CO_2 in the body as a result of failure of pulmonary ventilation. This itself may occur after lesions either in the central nervous system (e.g. depression of cerebral function, spinal cord injury) or in peripheral nervous pathways involved in ventilating the lungs (peripheral nerve and muscle disorders), or in some forms of lung disease involving impaired gas diffusion.

The decrease in body fluid pH resulting from carbonic acid generation is initially buffered to a limited extent by the reaction of carbonic acid with intracellular buffers such as haemoglobin, leading to the release of small amounts of bicarbonate into the plasma. However, longer term restoration of body fluid pH balance requires the excretion by the kidney of the net acid retained during the period of hypoventilation.

This is achieved by the three steps described above, namely total reabsorption of filtered bicarbonate, titration of all available filtered buffers, and increased generation of ammonia within the kidney to allow for a higher-than-baseline level of net acid excretion as ammonium ion. This latter step is stimulated both by intracellular acidosis and by the elevated pCO_2 which is associated with respiratory acidosis. Over a few days, a new steady state is achieved in which renal excretion of net acid matches that being retained by the lungs, the urine pH being low and the plasma bicarbonate being raised above baseline values (Fig. 4.5).

Metabolic acidosis

Metabolic acidosis (or, more correctly, non-respiratory acidosis), on the other hand, is associated with the accumulation of non-volatile acid within the body. There are essentially three components to the protective response which limits the fall in pH which would otherwise occur.

Physicochemical buffering
The first defence against a fall in the pH of the body fluids after addition of an acid load is the buffering of H^+ by available bases, particularly bicarbonate which is abundant in the ECF. This results in a fall in the plasma bicarbonate, and hence a lesser fall in the plasma pH

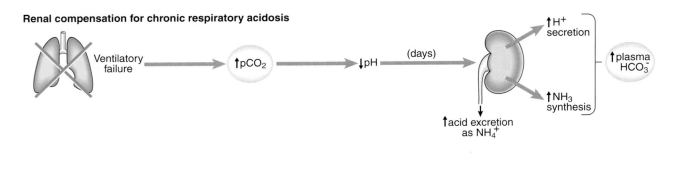

Renal compensation for chronic respiratory acidosis

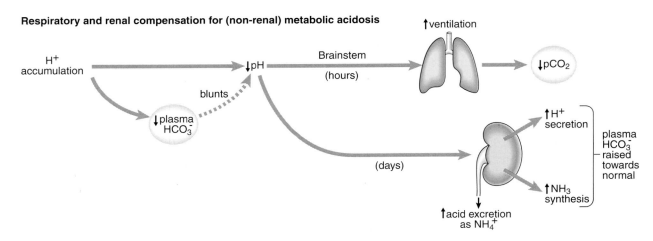

Respiratory and renal compensation for (non-renal) metabolic acidosis

Fig. 4.5
Mechanisms of renal and respiratory compensation for acid–base disturbances. The immediate action of physicochemical buffers is omitted for clarity.

than would otherwise have occurred. A variety of extracellular and intracellular proteins provide a further reserve of H^+ binding sites, and a limited amount of tissue phosphate also contributes some buffer capacity. These reactions are essentially complete within a few minutes of addition of acid to the body fluids, though further buffering occurs in bone and other tissues over the ensuing hours and days.

Respiratory response
Despite initial buffering, the pH of the plasma will still fall somewhat during acidosis, and this acts as a potent stimulus to increase the ventilation rate via the activation of chemoreceptors within the brainstem (ventral medulla) which respond to a fall in pH of the cerebrospinal fluid. Clinically this manifests as a deep, rapid breathing pattern (Kussmaul respiration). Over a matter of minutes to hours, this response drives the CO_2 below normal, and thus serves to blunt the fall in ECF pH by shifting the carbonic acid equilibrium reaction (see Fig. 4.1). This respiratory response provides a medium-term compensation for the acidosis produced by the metabolic disturbance. Note that while the resulting plasma pH is brought up towards 7.40, it

is not fully normalized, and never 'overshoots', as a result of respiratory compensation alone.

Renal response
Steady state correction of the acid–base disturbance requires the development over several days of an increased capacity by the kidney to excrete the metabolic acid load. This involves reabsorption of all filtered bicarbonate, maximum titration of filtered buffers with secreted H^+, and increased intrarenal synthesis of ammonia, which combines with secreted hydrogen ions in the luminal compartment and appears in the urine as large quantities of ammonium. The urine pH falls to minimum levels (around 4.5) and the plasma bicarbonate, lowered initially by the reaction with added acid and subsequently by the hyperventilation response, is elevated back up into the normal range. The net result is a restoration of plasma pH to normal.

Before leaving the subject of renal acid secretion, a number of factors which have been identified as regulators of this process should be listed. The principal factors causing an increase in H^+ secretion by the nephron include:

Acid–base balance and regulation of pH box 2

The arterial blood gases

Returning to the case of Mrs Loy, crucial early data needed to clarify her acid–base status are the pH and pCO_2 of the arterial blood. These are obtained immediately after her admission to hospital, and give the following results:

pH 7.37
*pCO_2 22 mmHg
*HCO_3^- 13 mmol/L
pO_2 103 mmHg.

These data confirm that her problem is primarily an acidosis (pH < 7.40) of metabolic origin (low HCO_3^-) which has undergone a considerable degree of respiratory compensation (low pCO_2). However, the presence of the low bicarbonate concentration implies that the kidney has not achieved long-term correction of the underlying acid accumulation.

The question now arises: what is the source of the metabolic acid load that is playing a major part in this presentation?

Before completing an analysis of her acid–base problem, we might take note of one clue present in the data available already. Whatever the cause of metabolic acid build-up, there is some problem with kidney function in this case since urinalysis showed a pH of 7. According to the description above of an expected renal response to acidosis involving excretion of a maximally acidic urine (pH < 5), the urine pH in this case is quite inappropriate and would appear to point to a primary problem located within the kidney itself. As will be seen, this was indeed the case.

- increase in filtered load of bicarbonate
- decrease in ECF volume
- decrease in plasma pH
- increase in blood pCO_2
- hypokalaemia
- aldosterone.

Note that the first two factors listed result in increased proximal bicarbonate reabsorption, while the later factors act in distal nephron segments to enhance net acid excretion. The common mediator in the case of the last four factors is probably a decrease in the intracellular pH of the tubular cells, which not only activates the hydrogen ion secretory mechanism but also enhances tubular ammonia synthesis.

See box 2.

Patterns of metabolic acidosis

Two basic types of metabolic acidosis can be distinguished, on the basis of the effect they have on readily measurable plasma parameters. In one type, acid might be added as hydrochloric (mineral) acid, or there might be a primary loss of bicarbonate buffer from the ECF. In this pattern, there is no addition to the plasma of a new acid anion. In the second type, the accumulating acid might be in the form of an organic acid where the acid anion accumulates in the plasma to replace the falling bicarbonate.

These concepts are shown in diagrammatic form in Fig. 4.6. When the concentrations of the commonly measured cations in the blood (sodium and potassium) are added, there is in normal plasma an apparent discrepancy of some 15 mmol/L over and above the sum of the two commonly measured anions (chloride and bicarbonate). This 'anion gap' is largely explained by the multiple negative charges on plasma protein molecules. It can be seen that, where mineral acid is added or bicarbonate is lost (pattern A), the fall in plasma bicarbonate is compensated by a rise in chloride, resulting in no change in the apparent anion gap. In pattern B, however, the bicarbonate may fall to the same extent, but this is accounted for by the addition of the organic acid anion, which, being itself unmeasured, adds to the apparent anion gap, and the plasma chloride does not change from normal. This simple analysis provides an initial tool for the diagnosis of the cause of a metabolic acidosis, where this is not obvious.

Some causes of normal anion gap metabolic acidosis are given in Table 4.1. Rarely, the cause is addition of hydrochloric acid or ammonium chloride, usually in a setting of medical investigation or treatment. More commonly, there is a problem either in the gastrointestinal tract involving loss of bicarbonate from the lower bowel, or in the kidney. In the latter case, the normal mechanisms for H^+ secretion into the lumen of the nephron may be impaired, either in the proximal tubule (such as by the carbonic anhydrase inhibitor acetazolamide), or in the distal nephron (where the processes involved in urinary acidification are defective). As a group, these disorders of renal acid excretion are called renal tubular acidoses, and will be discussed further later in this chapter.

Causes of the increased anion gap pattern of metabolic acidosis are given in Table 4.2. The organic acid load in these conditions may be classified as to whether it is of endogenous or exogenous origin. In some cases, when specifically suspected, such as lactate in lactic acidosis, the organic acid anion can be measured in the blood. In other cases, however, the

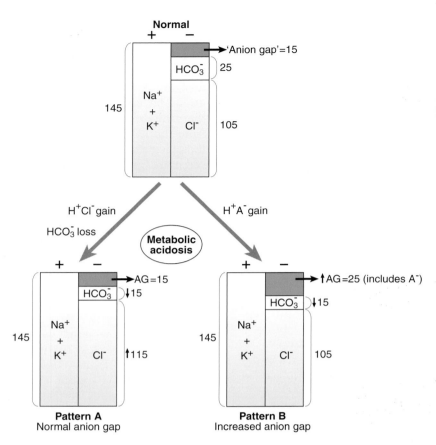

Fig. 4.6
Patterns of metabolic acidosis. All figures are in mmol/L. AG, anion gap.

clinical history provides a strong clue as to the cause, e.g. the accumulation of ketoacids in diabetic ketoacidosis, or of salicylate following aspirin intoxication (this latter disorder being complicated by respiratory alkalosis because of ventilatory stimulation). Of note is the predisposition of alcoholic patients to a number of forms of increased anion gap metabolic acidosis. These include starvation ketosis, lactic acidosis and intoxication by methanol or ethylene glycol (when consumed as alternatives to alcohol). Where metabolic acidosis is associated with advanced renal failure, the cause is usually the accumulation of complex organic acids normally excreted by filtration and proximal tubular secretion, and the result is an increased anion gap.

See box 3.

Renal tubular acidosis

Metabolic acidosis can arise as a result of failure of renal tubular segments to secrete hydrogen ions in the absence of any major impairment of glomerular filtration rate. This acidosis of renal tubular origin is

Table 4.1
Causes of normal anion gap metabolic acidosis

Disorder	Mechanism
Inorganic acid addition:	
Infusion/ingestion of HCl, NH_4Cl	Exogenous acid load
Gastrointestinal base loss:	
*Diarrhoea	Loss of bicarbonate from gut
Small bowel fistula/drainage	Loss of bicarbonate from gut
Surgical diversion of urine into gut loops	Secretion of $KHCO_3$ by bowel mucosa
Renal base loss/acid retention:	
Proximal renal tubular acidosis	Renal tubular bicarbonate wasting
Distal renal tubular acidosis	Impaired renal tubular acid secretion

*Diarrhoea alone is rarely associated with marked acidosis unless it is severe and prolonged.

not associated with accumulation of any organic acid anion, and so the anion gap remains normal. Two basic variants of the condition, which can be either congenital or acquired, are described.

Table 4.2
Causes of increased anion gap metabolic acidosis

Disorder	Anion(s)	Clues to diagnosis
Endogenous acid load:		
Diabetic ketoacidosis	Acetoacetate, beta-OH butyrate	Hyperglycaemia, ketonuria
Starvation ketosis	Acetoacetate, beta-OH butyrate	Hypoglycaemia
Lactic acidosis	Lactate	Shock, hypoxia, liver disease
Renal failure	Organic acids	Reduced glomerular filtration rate
Exogenous acid load:		
Salicylate poisoning	Salicylate	Associated with respiratory alkalosis
Methanol poisoning	Formate	Visual complaints, often alcoholic
Ethylene glycol poisoning	Glycolate, oxalate	Oxalate crystalluria, often alcoholic

Acid–base balance and regulation of pH box 3

The diagnosis

Mrs Loy's electrolyte profile was examined and an anion gap of 12 mmol/L was calculated (see original biochemistry data). There was no history of gastrointestinal disturbance and the urine pH was noted to be inappropriately high at 7. An interim diagnosis of renal tubular acidosis was made.

Further investigation, directed toward defining the immunological activity of her underlying connective tissue disease, revealed that the levels of **antinuclear antibodies** (including antibodies to double-stranded DNA) were elevated, and serum **complement** levels were low, consistent with activated SLE. In addition, the urine contained many red cells and red cell casts (see Chapter 7), and a large amount of protein. Renal biopsy confirmed severe diffuse inflammation affecting the glomeruli as well as the **tubulointerstitium**.

A diagnosis of reactivated SLE was made, with the complications of diffuse lupus nephritis (see Chapter 7) and renal tubular acidosis. The distal tubular dysfunction in this setting reflects a disruptive effect of the interstitial inflammatory changes on the transport properties of the tubules.

Table 4.3
Some causes of renal tubular acidosis (RTA)

Proximal RTA
Congenital (Fanconi syndrome, cystinosis, Wilson's disease)
Paraproteinaemia (e.g. myeloma)
Hyperparathyroidism
Drugs (carbonic anhydrase inhibitors)

Distal RTA ('classic' type)
Congenital
Hyperglobulinaemia
Autoimmune connective tissue diseases (e.g. systemic lupus erythematosus)
Toxins and drugs (toluene, lithium, amphotericin)

Hyperkalaemic distal RTA
Hypoaldosteronism
Obstructive nephropathy
Renal transplant rejection
Drugs (amiloride, spironolactone)

through later nephron segments. Plasma bicarbonate falls, blood pH falls, and bicarbonate appears in the urine.

- In distal RTA, the defect is in the late distal tubule and collecting duct segments, where acid secretion is mediated by an H^+-ATPase. In the classic form of this disorder, the hydrogen pump itself is probably defective. In other forms, such as that induced by amphotericin (an antifungal antibiotic), the impairment of net acid secretion results from back-leak of hydrogen ions across an epithelium which is made abnormally permeable to these ions.

Some causes of proximal and distal RTA are given in Table 4.3. Both proximal and distal RTA may be inherited as a primary defect, but a number of other conditions may produce secondary RTA in either segment. Notably, an alteration in proximal tubular function can be induced by high **paraprotein** levels as in **myeloma**, or by hyperparathyroidism, or by the carbonic anhydrase inhibitor acetazolamide. Distal

- In proximal renal tubular acidosis (RTA), the defect lies in the mechanism normally present within the proximal tubular epithelium for reabsorbing bicarbonate (refer to Fig. 4.2). Thus, either because of a specific defect in one of the components of the cellular acid secretory mechanism in this segment or because of non-specific damage to, or malfunction of, the proximal tubular epithelium as a whole, filtered bicarbonate is incompletely reabsorbed. This results in a large flow of bicarbonate, together with sodium,

RTA, on the other hand, can be caused by conditions associated with polyclonal **hyperglobulinaemia**, including SLE, as in the patient studied in this chapter. Other forms of structural tubulointerstitial disease can produce the same defect, and a number of drugs and toxins are also prone to damage this segment selectively.

Apart from the differences in clinical setting and aetiology between the proximal and distal types of RTA, a number of physiological differences exist. In the distal form, the impaired operation of the collecting duct H⁺ pump means that, no matter how severe the systemic acidosis, the urine pH can never be lowered appropriately, and generally remains above 5.5. Bicarbonate loss is not prominent since proximal reabsorption is generally intact. However, in early or mild forms of proximal RTA there is considerable leak of bicarbonate into the urine, which again has an inappropriately high pH since the distal segments are unable to acidify the urine as long as large amounts of bicarbonate are flooding through the lumen from the proximal segments. However, when acidosis is more severe in proximal RTA, the plasma bicarbonate falls because of buffering of the accumulated acid. As a result, a point may be reached where the reduced filtered amount of bicarbonate can be largely reabsorbed by the defective proximal tubular reabsorptive mechanism. The intact distal segments can then reabsorb a small distal leak of bicarbonate, as normally occurs. In this situation the distal tubular secretory pump can operate normally and generate a transtubular H⁺ concentration gradient, resulting in a lowering of the final urine pH. When this occurs, bicarbonate loss ceases and ammonium excretion rises so that a new steady state arises in which acid retention stabilizes, albeit at a reduced plasma bicarbonate concentration.

There are also differences in some of the associated features of proximal *versus* distal RTA. The proximal type may be associated with loss of other molecules normally reabsorbed in the proximal tubule, giving rise to amino aciduria, glycosuria and phosphaturia. A different problem occurs in distal RTA as a result of progressive accumulation of acid over many years. As a consequence of buffering of H⁺ in bone, calcium is released from the skeleton and may be deposited in the tissues, including the kidney (nephrocalcinosis). Furthermore, the high urinary excretion of calcium may result in stone formation (see Chapter 10), often associated with urinary tract infection. Impairment of skeletal growth can occur in this condition, and also in proximal RTA when the disorder is congenital or starts in early childhood.

Much of the symptomatology of both kinds of RTA relates to electrolyte depletion. Urinary losses of sodium are abnormally high in both forms, resulting in a degree of hypovolaemia. Both forms are typically also associated with hypokalaemia because of stimulated potassium secretion in the late distal and cortical collecting ducts. This is caused by a high luminal flow of sodium and bicarbonate in proximal RTA, and by electrically-driven potassium secretion to replace faulty H⁺ secretion in distal RTA.

An important variant of distal RTA is hyperkalaemic distal RTA (sometimes called type 4 RTA). In this case the normal anion gap metabolic acidosis is associated with hyperkalaemia, which points to a different site of defect in the acid-secreting segment of the nephron. As shown in Fig. 4.7, if a disruption occurs in the normal

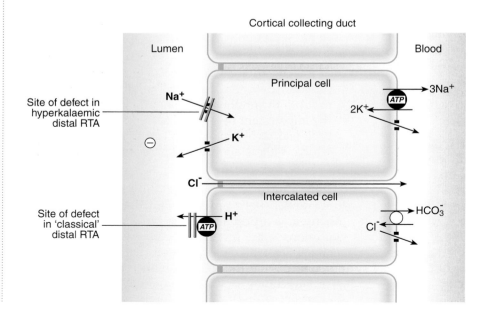

Fig. 4.7
Site of defect in two variants of distal renal tubular acidosis (RTA).

operation of the principal cell type in this tubular segment, sodium reabsorption will be impaired, resulting in a loss of the normal lumen negativity (see Chapter 2). This electrical change impairs the rate of secretion of both potassium and hydrogen ions into the lumen, resulting in systemic acidosis with hyperkalaemia. This lesion has been described in a variety of conditions causing distal tubulointerstitial damage (such as urinary tract obstruction with infection), and also during treatment with drugs interfering with principal cell sodium transport (such as amiloride). A similar defect results from deficiencies in aldosterone secretion or action, including diseases of the adrenal cortex and of the renin secretory mechanism in the kidney.

The management of all forms of RTA is directed in the first instance toward reversing the underlying condition affecting tubular function, if possible. The next principle is that sufficient bicarbonate buffer must be provided to replace that consumed by the acid being accumulated. Provision of some of this bicarbonate as potassium salt will help replete potassium lost in classic forms of the disorder, while in the hyperkalaemic variant of distal RTA, measures to assist in the excretion of potassium (e.g. loop or thiazide diuretics, or corticosteroids, as appropriate) may be necessary. Treatment may also be required for specific complications in the various forms of the condition, such as removal of stones and treatment of infections which sometimes complicate classic distal RTA.

Acid–base balance and regulation of pH box 4

Treatment and outcome

Mrs Loy's treatment focused on the control of her underlying connective tissue disease. Immunosuppression using prednisone and cyclophosphamide was initiated with a view to reducing the activity of her SLE. The metabolic acidosis and hypokalaemia were corrected initially with infusions, and later with oral supplements, of alkaline salts of sodium and potassium.

Over the ensuing weeks her condition improved dramatically, with the fevers and rash subsiding, urinary protein and red cell excretion reduced, and plasma electrolyte profile reverted towards normal. Within several weeks it was possible to discontinue her electrolyte and buffer therapy, and ongoing management was directed towards long-term stabilization of the connective tissue disease.

Disturbances of acid–base balance: alkalosis

To complete our survey of acid–base disturbances, we can consider the two primary perturbations which might result in alkalosis.

Respiratory alkalosis

Any form of sustained hyperventilation will produce a reduction in the blood pCO_2 with a resulting increase in plasma pH. The respiratory stimulus most commonly arises from anxiety states, but it may also be due to drugs stimulating the respiratory centre, other brain disorders and chronic liver disease.

The homeostatic response to respiratory alkalosis involves an initial phase of physicochemical buffering by intracellular proteins, which give up H^+, resulting in a small decrease in the plasma bicarbonate. More sustained compensation occurs over the ensuing days, during which renal tubular H^+ secretion is inhibited by the high extracellular pH and the reduced pCO_2. Bicarbonate reabsorption is inhibited, as is ammonium excretion, and the result is a reduction in net acid excretion and a fall in the plasma bicarbonate. In many cases the respiratory disturbance is not unduly prolonged, and the renal compensation subsides as ventilation is normalized.

Metabolic alkalosis

In this disorder there is a primary increase in the plasma bicarbonate concentration and the plasma pH. The causes fall into two groups according to whether there is associated contraction of the ECF volume or not.

Hypovolaemic metabolic alkalosis is the commonest pattern, and includes disorders such as vomiting and gastric suction, in which acid-rich gastric juices are lost from the body. Metabolic alkalosis associated with volume contraction also occurs during treatment with most diuretics (other than carbonic anhydrase inhibitors and potassium-sparing drugs). Here there is increased acid loss into the urine related to the diuretic action on the tubules. The alkalosis associated with volume contraction is perpetuated by secondary renal responses, described in more detail below.

Normovolaemic (or hypervolaemic) metabolic alkalosis occurs when the primary disturbance provokes both bicarbonate retention and a degree of volume expansion. This most commonly occurs in corticosteroid excess states such as primary hyperaldosteronism (Conn's syndrome), Cushing's syndrome and related disorders. Occasionally, overuse of antacid salts can produce a similar pattern.

The homeostatic response to metabolic alkalosis involves initial buffering of the rise in plasma bicarbonate by titration of extracellular and intracellular buffers, including plasma proteins. Soon afterwards, the increased pH acts to inhibit ventilation through the medullary chemoreceptors, such that the pCO_2 starts to rise. Since, however, this is ultimately associated with an unacceptable degree of hypoxia, the extent to which this form of compensation occurs is limited, such that the maximum pCO_2 attained is rarely more than 55 mmHg.

In the absence of counterbalancing stimuli, the expected renal response to sustained metabolic alkalosis would be to decrease tubular acid secretion, inhibit bicarbonate reabsorption and excrete the excess bicarbonate into the urine. However, in the commonest form of metabolic alkalosis, that caused by sustained vomiting, this response is distorted by other changes associated with the loss of gastric fluid. As shown in Fig. 4.8, the loss of H^+ initiates the alkalosis ('generation' phase), which is actually worsened by the losses of sodium, water and potassium ('maintenance' phase). The sodium losses are associated with hypovolaemia, which triggers both proximal bicarbonate reabsorption and aldosterone release, which stimulates distal acid secretion, thereby aggravating the systemic alkalosis. Furthermore, the hypokalaemia resulting from potassium loss (more through the kidney than from gastric fluid) also stimulates distal acid secretion and tubular ammonia synthesis (see earlier), both of which enhance acid excretion and maintain the alkalosis. The net result is an inappropriately acid urine and a failure of the kidney to effect long-term correction of the systemic pH disturbance.

The cornerstone of management in hypovolaemic metabolic alkalosis states, exemplified by vomiting, is to provide adequate volume replacement as sodium chloride (isotonic saline infusions), which switches off the volume-conserving mechanisms mentioned above and allows the kidney to excrete the excess alkali in the urine. Replacement of potassium helps correct the hypokalaemia and its consequences in the kidney.

The non-hypovolaemic forms of metabolic alkalosis, by way of contrast, are resistant to treatment with sodium chloride, but can usually be managed by cessation of alkali therapy or correction of mineralocorticoid excess. The latter may involve either adrenal gland surgery or blockade of mineralocorticoid effect in the kidney by treatment with spironolactone.

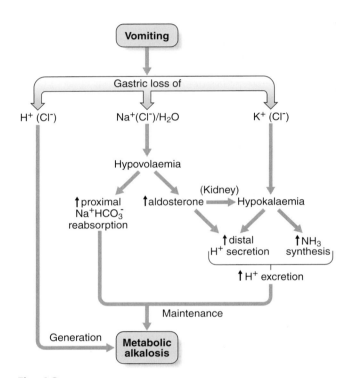

Fig. 4.8
Vomiting: generation and maintenance of metabolic alkalosis. Note that the gastric loss of H^+ is primarily responsible for generating the systemic alkalosis, while the other mechanisms shown act through the kidney to maintain the alkalosis as long as sodium and potassium losses are uncorrected. Chloride is the deficient anion accompanying all cations shown.

Table 4.4
Summary of 'simple' acid–base disturbances

Disorder	pH	Primary change	Compensatory response
Metabolic acidosis	Decreased	Decreased HCO_3^-	Decreased pCO_2
Metabolic alkalosis	Increased	Increased HCO_3^-	Increased pCO_2
Respiratory acidosis	Decreased	Increased pCO_2	Increased HCO_3^-
Respiratory alkalosis	Increased	Decreased pCO_2	Decreased HCO_3^-

Summary of findings in principal acid–base disturbances

Table 4.4 provides an overview of the changes in pH, bicarbonate concentration and pCO_2 in the four major simple acid–base disorders. Taken in conjunction with clinical information, the results of these analyses are usually sufficient to enable a diagnosis to be made of the nature and cause of the disturbance. Rules of thumb are available to indicate the predicted compensatory change in pCO_2 or bicarbonate levels expected in each of the simple (uncomplicated) acid–base disorders. When the available data for a given patient are not consistent with these changes, a complex or 'mixed' acid–base disorder can be inferred, and the elements of the disturbance usually deduced in conjunction with a thorough clinical evaluation.

Self-assessment case study

A consultation is requested on an 81-year-old man who has been admitted to the hospital with an acute myocardial infarction (heart attack). There has been significant damage to the left ventricle such that cardiac output is markedly reduced. Furthermore, on day 5 after admission his course is complicated by the development of acute ischaemia in the left leg, attributed to occlusion of a major leg artery following embolization of a thrombus from the left ventricular cavity.

The patient's plasma electrolyte results are as follows:

Sodium 135 mmol/L
*Potassium 5.2 mmol/L
Chloride 97 mmol/L
*Bicarbonate 14 mmol/L
*Urea 14.0 mmol/L
*Creatinine 0.14 mmol/L.
(*Values outside normal range; see Appendix.)

Arterial blood gas analysis reveal the following: pH 7.33, pCO_2 29 mmHg, pO_2 (breathing room air) 58 mmHg.

After studying this chapter you should be able to answer the following questions:

① What is the overall pattern of acid–base disturbance in this patient?

② What is the anion gap in this patient?

③ What is the likely cause of the disturbance in this case?

④ What would you expect the urine pH to be?

⑤ What are the principles of treatment?

⑥ What would the effect of a bicarbonate infusion be on his plasma potassium concentration?

Answers see page 146

Self-assessment questions

① What would the effect on systemic acid–base balance be if a patient were given long-term treatment with a carbonic anhydrase inhibitor such as acetazolamide?

② Where in the nephron is the steepest gradient of pH between the plasma and the luminal fluid?

③ Name three changes in the plasma which stimulate an increase in hydrogen ion secretion by the nephron.

④ Give three causes of a metabolic acidosis with a normal anion gap.

⑤ Name three factors which perpetuate the systemic alkalosis which follows prolonged vomiting.

Answers see page 146

GLOMERULAR FILTRATION AND ACUTE RENAL FAILURE

Chapter objectives

After studying this chapter you should be able to:

① Define the determinants of renal blood flow and glomerular filtration.

② Describe the mechanism of glomerular filtration.

③ Understand the factors that govern autoregulation within the kidney.

④ Understand the concept of clearance and be familiar with the different methods of assessment of renal function.

⑤ Determine whether oliguria is physiological or due to established renal failure.

⑥ Recognize the clinical circumstances in which acute renal failure is likely to occur.

⑦ Describe the cellular and biochemical mechanisms which underlie acute renal failure caused by acute tubular necrosis.

⑧ Outline a logical clinical, laboratory and radiological approach to the assessment of a patient presenting with renal failure.

⑨ Define the acute clinical complications and the biochemical and haematological abnormalities in acute renal failure.

⑩ Effectively anticipate, prevent and treat the complications occurring in acute renal failure.

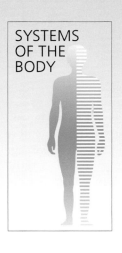

SYSTEMS
OF THE
BODY

Introduction

As described in previous chapters, the primary functions of the kidney are to maintain body fluid, electrolyte and acid–base homeostasis, and to excrete nitrogenous wastes. These functions rely on a normal anatomical outflow pathway, a normal renal circulation, and normal intrarenal mechanisms for regulating the process of urine formation. Abnormalities in any of these structures or processes can underlie the development of acute renal failure, characterized by an abrupt fall in glomerular filtration rate (GFR). After studying this chapter you should be able to describe the mechanism of glomerular filtration, the factors normally involved in its regulation, and the causes, consequences and treatment of acute renal failure.

See box 1.

Renal blood flow

Renal blood flow is between 1.0 and 1.2 litres per minute per $1.73\,m^2$ of body surface area. The majority of blood flow to the kidney is directed to the cortex, with only a small proportion delivered to the medulla, where sodium transport by the thick ascending limb of the loop of Henle accounts for a high oxygen consumption. Thus the renal medulla is sensitive to reductions in renal blood flow and oxygen delivery that may induce hypoxia and result in tubular damage, causing acute renal failure.

The main determinant of the overall renal blood flow is the state of vasoconstriction of the renal arterial tree. Changes in the intrarenal vascular resistance mediate significant alterations in renal blood flow under pathophysiological conditions, while over a wide range of physiological mean arterial pressure levels, renal vasoregulation contributes to the maintenance of a stable renal blood flow and hence GFR (see below, under Autoregulation).

Glomerular filtration

As described earlier in this book, the key process involved in the kidney's excretory function is the formation of an ultrafiltrate of plasma in the glomeruli, where capillary tufts arising from the arterial circulation meet the blind ends of the tubular system in which urine is modified and conducted into the urine drainage system.

The structure of the glomerulus will be discussed in detail in Chapter 6. In brief, the process of filtration occurs across a complex barrier consisting of the thin **fenestrated** endothelial lining of the glomerular capil-

Glomerular filtration and acute renal failure box 1

A presentation with anuria

Joan Wood is a 60-year-old woman who presented to the Emergency Department with a 4-day history of abdominal pain and vomiting, during which she had been unable to tolerate any food or fluids orally. She had passed no urine in the last 24 h.

Her past history included poorly controlled hypertension, with current treatment being an angiotensin-converting enzyme inhibitor (ramipril 10 mg/day), a loop diuretic (furosemide; frusemide 40 mg/day), and a dihydropyridine calcium channel blocker (amlodipine 5 mg/day).

Clinically she was febrile at 38.6°C. Her blood pressure was 100/60 mmHg with a postural drop of 10 mmHg. She was tachycardic, with a pulse rate of 100 beats/min. Her jugular venous pressure was only just visible lying flat and her mucous membranes were dry. Her abdomen was distended, with tenderness in the left iliac fossa and an ill defined mass was present. Bowel sounds were absent, consistent with bowel obstruction.

Bladder catheterization yielded 50 ml of urine, and urinalysis showed protein trace, blood trace and specific gravity 1015.

Clinical evaluation and computed tomography (CT) scanning suggested that the likely diagnosis was **diverticular disease** complicated by an abscess, resulting in systemic sepsis.

This patient is clearly critically unwell, with sepsis and dehydration arising from a surgical disorder of the bowel. The failure to pass urine in this setting (anuria) is a crucial element of the presentation, suggesting the development of impaired renal excretory function and a reduced GFR.

This scenario gives rise to the questions:

① What is the mechanism of glomerular filtration, and how is it normally regulated?

② How can the cause of an abnormally low rate of urine production be determined?

lary, the glomerular basement membrane, and the foot processes of the epithelial cells (derived from the end of the tubular system) apposed to the external wall of the capillary. This filtration barrier allows free passage of solutes (up to a molecular weight of around 60000 D), but retains cells and protein within the circulation. The selective properties of this barrier, and the consequences of its disruption, will be discussed further in the next two chapters.

The filtration process itself is based on purely passive forces, of which the hydrostatic pressure generated by the heart is the principal driving force. However, as shown in Fig. 5.1, this outward filtration pressure is partially opposed by two pressures acting to restrain filtration, namely the hydrostatic pressure within the lumen of the tubular system itself, and by the oncotic pressure due to plasma proteins which are retained within the capillary. Thus the net ultrafiltration pressure (P_{uf}) comprises the hydrostatic pressure in the glomerular capillaries (P_{gc}) minus the hydrostatic pressure in the tubules (P_t) minus the oncotic pressure generated by plasma proteins (π_{gc}).

An overall expression for GFR which indicates all of its determinants is as follows:

$$GFR = K_f \times P_{uf}$$

where K_f is the ultrafiltration coefficient, which is made up of the product of the hydraulic permeability of the filtration membrane times the surface area available for filtration.

Typical mean values for the pressure terms indicate that: $P_{gc} = 45\,mmHg$, $P_t = 10\,mmHg$, $\pi_{gc} = 25\,mmHg$, giving rise to a net ultrafiltration pressure P_{uf} of $10\,mmHg$.

Factors which interfere with any of these determinants of glomerular filtration may lead to an abrupt fall in GFR and thus acute renal failure unless adequate compensatory responses occur. The most important physiological determinant is the capillary hydrostatic pressure, which may be reduced either by a reduction in perfusion pressure reaching the afferent arteriole, by an increase in afferent arteriolar tone, or by a decrease in efferent arteriolar tone (see below). The pressure in the tubular system may rise significantly during ureteric obstruction, thus reducing the GFR. Changes in the plasma oncotic pressure are less important in altering GFR under physiological or pathological conditions. Pathological change involving the glomeruli may lead to alterations in the ultrafiltration coefficient by decreasing the hydraulic permeability and/or by obliterating the total capillary surface area available for filtration. Conditions such as glomerulonephritis (see Chapter 7) and diabetes mellitus (see Chapter 8) impair glomerular filtration by these mechanisms.

Under physiological conditions, the regulation of the filtration rate in individual glomeruli is determined by the balance between the resistance in the afferent and efferent arterioles. As shown in Fig. 5.2, the hydrostatic pressure across the wall of the glomerular capillaries will be increased by factors either dilating the afferent arteriole, or constricting the efferent arteriole, increasing the single nephron GFR in either case. Conversely, factors leading to afferent arteriolar constriction or efferent arteriolar dilatation will reduce the filtration rate of the affected glomerulus. Some circulating substances known to have these effects are shown in Fig. 5.2. It should be noted, however, that in the normal kidney minor perturbations in levels of individual substances do not have significant net effects on GFR because of compensatory changes in other factors which tend to maintain a haemodynamic steady state. However, if renal function is impaired, particularly because of a low renal perfusion pressure (e.g. renal artery stenosis or cardiac failure), maintenance of GFR is highly dependent on intrinsic compensatory mechanisms such as afferent arteriolar vasodilatation (predominantly due to prostaglandins) and efferent arteriolar vasoconstriction (predominantly due to angiotensin II). Thus, factors which interfere with these compensatory mechanisms, such as non-steroidal anti-inflammatory drugs (which inhibit prostaglandin synthesis) and angiotensin-converting enzyme inhibitors or angiotensin II receptor blockers (which interfere with angiotensin II action), blunt these compensatory responses and may precipitate acute renal failure (see Chapter 11).

It should be noted that angiotensin II has a particularly important but complex role in the regulation of glomerular filtration. While local production of this

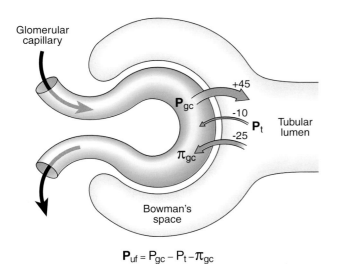

$$\mathbf{P}_{uf} = \mathbf{P}_{gc} - \mathbf{P}_t - \pi_{gc}$$

Fig. 5.1

Diagram of glomerulus showing the forces involved in glomerular filtration. P_{uf}, net ultrafiltration pressure; P_{gc}, hydrostatic pressure in glomerular capillary; P_t, hydrostatic pressure in tubular lumen; π_{gc}, oncotic pressure (osmotic pressure due to plasma proteins) in the glomerular capillary. Representative pressures are shown in mmHg.

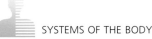

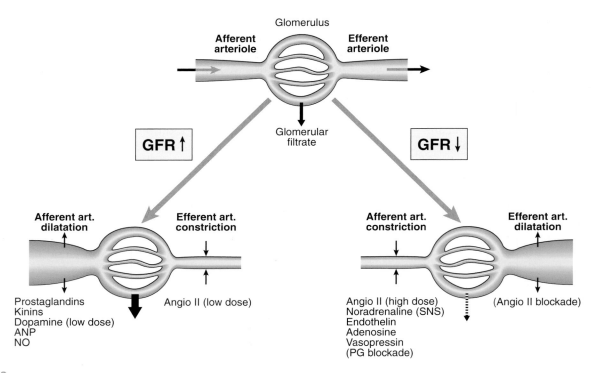

Fig. 5.2
Factors altering glomerular filtration rate (GFR) by changing the resistance in the afferent and efferent arterioles. ANP, atrial natriuretic peptide; Angio II, angiotensin II; NO, nitric oxide; PG, prostaglandin; SNS, sympathetic nervous system.

peptide acts predominantly on the efferent arteriole to maintain single nephron GFR, higher circulating levels are capable of producing afferent arteriolar vasoconstriction which tends to reduce glomerular filtration. Furthermore, angiotensin II causes contraction of the mesangial cells which support the glomerular capillary network, leading to a reduction in surface area available for filtration and so further acting to reduce filtration. The net effect in a particular physiological or pathophysiological circumstance depends on the balance between these actions, as well as other haemodynamic compensations which occur.

Autoregulation of renal blood flow and glomerular filtration rate

Renal blood flow is generally kept constant over a wide range of blood pressures. This phenomenon, called autoregulation, ensures constancy of glomerular filtration and thus solute excretion despite changes in systemic haemodynamics within certain limits (Fig. 5.3). While a variety of neural and vasoactive pathways may be involved in stabilizing the renal blood flow under these conditions, two particular mechanisms have been invoked to explain the autoregulation of GFR.

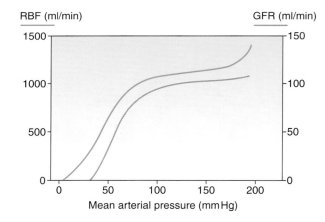

Fig. 5.3
Autoregulation of renal blood flow (RBF) and glomerular filtration rate (GFR).

First, the *myogenic mechanism* refers to the intrinsic capacity of afferent arteriolar smooth muscle cells to increase their state of contraction in response to an increase in renal perfusion pressure. This response, probably mediated by vasoactive agents produced by endothelial cells acting on smooth muscle cells in the afferent arteriole, serves to blunt the transmission of changed arteriolar pressure into the glomerular capillary bed.

The second mechanism is *tubuloglomerular feedback* (TGF). This describes the process whereby the GFR in individual nephrons is regulated according to the rate of solute flow through that nephron. As described in Chapter 2, the juxtaglomerular apparatus consists of a structure at which the distal tubule of a given nephron comes into close proximity with the afferent and efferent arterioles of the same nephron, where the tubular wall becomes specialized as the macula densa (Fig. 5.4; see also Fig. 2.10). Hence, the ionic composition (and indirectly, the flow rate) of the tubular fluid can be sensed by the macula densa, which signals directly to the vascular structures of the glomerulus to influence GFR. In brief, during conditions of avid tubular sodium chloride reabsorption, the sodium chloride concentration of the luminal fluid is reduced at the macula densa. Filtration in the corresponding glomerulus is increased, primarily by dilatation of the afferent arteriole. Conversely, when sodium chloride concentration and fluid delivery are high at the macula densa, afferent arteriolar tone is increased and single nephron GFR falls. This feedback mechanism, probably designed to limit the loss of fluid and electrolytes from damaged nephrons, also contributes to the

process of autoregulation. This is because increases in renal perfusion pressure would, of themselves, tend to lead to increased filtration and solute loss, which TGF effectively blunts. The mediator of the vasoconstrictor response involved in TGF appears to be locally produced adenosine, acting via the adenosine 1 receptor on the afferent arteriole. It is possible that other vasoactive mechanisms also play a part.

Renal excretion and the clearance formula

The rate at which a solute (s) is excreted by the kidney (E_s) is given simply by the product of the concentration of the solute in the urine (U_s) and the urine flow rate (V), which is the urine volume over a defined period. That is:

$$E_s = U_s \times V$$

where the units of E are mmol/min (or equivalent). This expression is useful in assessing absolute removal rates of solute by the kidney, and hence evaluating total body mass balance.

The renal clearance (C_s) of solute (s) on the other hand, is defined as the apparent volume of plasma from which the substance is completely removed per unit time during passage through the kidneys. It is equivalent mathematically to the ratio of the excretion rate to the simultaneous plasma concentration for that substance (P_s):

$$C_s = (U_s \times V)/P_s$$

The units of clearance are mL/min (or equivalent). The clearance calculation provides a measure of the relative efficiency of the kidney in removing a given solute from the plasma, and a means of comparison between substances which are handled differently by the nephron. The range of possible clearance rates is from zero (for a substance which is either not filtered at all or is filtered and then completely reabsorbed by the tubular system) up to a maximum equivalent to the renal plasma flow rate (for a substance which is filtered and totally secreted by the tubular system). Interpretation of clearance calculations depends on knowing whether the substance is freely filtered at the glomerulus. The procedure requires the presence of a steady state in the plasma concentration throughout the time frame of the period under study.

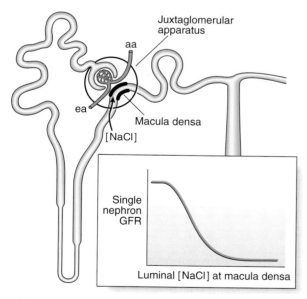

Fig. 5.4
Tubuloglomerular feedback. [NaCl] refers to the concentration of NaCl in the luminal fluid at the macula densa (top of the ascending limb of the loop of Henle). The inset shows the shape of the relationship between the [NaCl] at the macula densa and the glomerular filtration rate (GFR) in the same nephron.

Measuring the glomerular filtration rate

The utility of the clearance concept in renal physiology is illustrated best by its application to the determination of GFR. As shown in Fig. 5.5, the renal handling

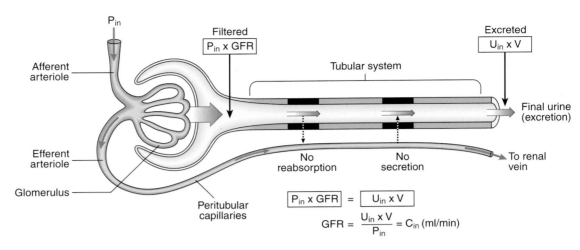

Fig. 5.5
Schematic illustration of the application of the clearance concept to the determination of the glomerular filtration rate (GFR). P_{in}, inulin concentration in plasma brought to the glomerulus; U_{in}, inulin concentration in final urine; V, urine flow rate; C_{in}, clearance of inulin.

of the plant polysaccharide inulin is such that it is freely filtered at the glomerulus and undergoes no reabsorption or secretion during its passage through the tubular system. It follows from simple mass balance that the amount being filtered into the early part of the tubular system equals the amount being excreted at the end of that system. As shown in Fig. 5.5, this gives rise to the inference that the GFR can be measured by determining the clearance of inulin, which is possible experimentally simply by measuring its concentration in the plasma and urine, as well as the urine flow rate, during a steady state infusion.

Unfortunately, there are logistical difficulties involved in determining inulin clearance since it needs to be infused and is difficult to assay. While a variety of other substances behave in a way similar to inulin and can be used clinically (e.g. iothalamate), in practice a great advantage is gained by using the clearance of an endogenous molecule whose behaviour approximates that of inulin for clinical determination of GFR. Such a substance is creatinine, derived from the metabolic breakdown of creatine, a component of skeletal muscle. For a given individual, the amount of creatinine entering the circulation per day is dependent almost exclusively on the skeletal muscle mass. As long as renal function is stable, this same daily amount will be excreted in the urine, given by the product of U_{cr} and V. Creatinine, like inulin, is freely filtered at the glomerulus and undergoes no tubular reabsorption, although there is a small degree of secretion by the tubules when renal function is impaired. None the less, under most conditions the clearance of endogenous creatinine provides a measure of GFR which is suffi-

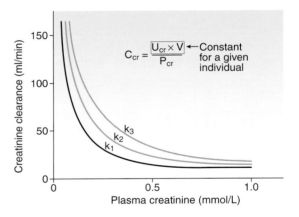

Fig. 5.6
Relationship between creatinine clearance (an estimate of glomerular filtration rate) and plasma creatinine concentration. C_{cr}, creatinine clearance; U_{cr}, urine creatinine concentration; V, urine flow rate; P_{cr}, plasma creatinine concentration. k_1 represents the curve for a small–average patient, while k_2 and k_3 show the position of the curve for progressively heavier patients.

ciently robust for clinical use. Moreover, because $U_{cr} \times V$ is a constant for a given individual under steady state conditions, there is a fixed relationship between the GFR and plasma creatinine, in the form of a rectangular hyperbola as shown in Fig. 5.6.

Several important deductions can be made from inspection of this relationship. First, plasma creatinine only starts to increase substantially when approximately 50% of renal function (GFR) is lost. Thus, a significant reduction in GFR can be present before the plasma creatinine is recorded outside the 'normal' reference range for a laboratory. Second, each such relationship is specific to a given individual with a particular muscle mass, making comparison of plasma creatinine between patients of different morphology difficult. For example, in patients with a low muscle mass, particularly elderly females, plasma creatinine can lie within the normal range in the presence of marked reductions in renal function. This is equivalent to saying that patients with increasing muscle masses have different GFR *versus* plasma creatinine graphs, displaced to the right in Fig. 5.6 for increasing muscle mass.

To obviate some of these difficulties in interpretation of plasma creatinine, a number of nomograms have been devised which give a reasonably accurate estimate of GFR from the plasma creatinine in an individual of a certain age, weight and sex. The best known such relationship is that of Cockcroft and Gault, namely:

$$\text{Estimated GFR (mL/min)}$$
$$= \frac{(140 - \text{age}) \times \text{weight (kg)}}{814 \times \text{plasma creatinine (mmol/L)}}$$

The result should be multiplied by 0.85 for women to allow for the relatively lower proportion of body weight which is muscle.

Urea

Urea is one of the main metabolic products of protein metabolism, and its excretion into the urine is one of the key functions of the kidney. Urea ($NH_2.CO.NH_2$) is synthesized in the liver from ammonium ions, derived from amino acid catabolism, plus carbon dioxide. It is freely filtered at the glomerulus, but undergoes approximately 50% reabsorption during passage through the nephron. Thus the clearance of urea is approximately half the GFR, and plasma urea varies inversely with the GFR. However, the fraction of filtered urea which is reabsorbed is not constant, being greater during conditions of dehydration and low urine flow rate. This makes urea less valuable as a direct measure of GFR than creatinine, since it is influenced not only by the GFR but also by the state of hydration. Furthermore, urea production is related to the amount of protein absorbed from the gut and to the protein catabolic rate (Table 5.1). Consideration of the factors in this table allows for an informed interpretation of the results of plasma creatinine and urea levels. This will be of value later in our consideration of Mrs Wood.

Table 5.1

Factors causing an increase in plasma creatinine and urea concentrations

Creatinine	Urea
Decreased GFR	Decreased GFR
Increased skeletal muscle mass (long-term)	Decreased urine flow rate
	Increased protein intake:
	Diet
	Gastrointestinal bleeding
	Increased protein catabolic rate:
	Sepsis
	Steroid therapy
	Some tetracycline antibiotics

GFR, glomerular filtration rate.

Pathophysiology of oliguria

We turn now to a consideration of the origin and significance of the greatly reduced urine volume in the present patient. The urinary volume varies widely on a daily basis in normal individuals because of regulatory mechanisms aimed at maintaining a normal and constant body fluid volume. As described in Chapter 2, the main factors that are regulated to control body fluid volume and osmolality are the rates of reabsorption of sodium and water during their passage through the nephron. During states of sodium depletion and extracellular fluid (ECF) volume contraction, sodium reabsorptive mechanisms are activated, resulting in excretion of urine with a low sodium content. Similarly, during water deprivation, the kidney can concentrate urine sufficiently to maintain water balance at an intake of less than 500 mL/day. This capacity is largely related to the anatomical and physiological integrity of the tubular structures within the renal medulla, and their responsiveness to antidiuretic hormone, which is released during states of dehydration.

Thus, a low urine flow rate itself may be a normal response to hypovolaemia, often accompanied by systemic and renal haemodynamic changes ('prerenal' oliguria). By definition, acute renal failure is only present when there is evidence for a reduced GFR; indeed, this diagnosis can be made in the presence of a normal or even increased urine volume under certain circumstances. However, when there is sustained oliguria, defined as a urine volume of less than 400 mL/24 h, the likelihood of a low GFR is increased, but it is necessary to establish whether this is essentially 'physiological' and reversible, or pathological and indicative of structural renal damage.

The clinical history and examination are often helpful in suggesting which of these patterns of olig-

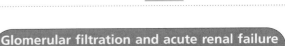
uria is present in a particular patient. Thus, sustained hypovolaemia or shock, or the presence of toxins known to cause tubular necrosis (see below), suggests that widespread damage to the parenchyma is likely, while shorter lived or lesser insults make 'physiological' oliguria more likely. A number of biochemical measurements have been found to provide assistance in making this differentiation. As shown in Table 5.2, markers of functional oliguria on a prerenal basis are those predicted by the expected physiological responses outlined above: thus urinary sodium concentration and fractional sodium excretion are low in this setting, but high when tubular damage is established. Osmolality and creatinine concentrations are high in the urine in prerenal oliguria, and low when damage is established. As predicted by the above discussion of factors influencing plasma urea and creatinine concentrations, the ratio of plasma urea to creatinine is high in prerenal oliguria, and lower in tubular necrosis.

In broad terms, the functional oliguria associated with physiological responses to hypovolaemia is reversible with appropriate fluid replacement therapy, while that associated with structural damage is less likely to be so. Thus, making this differentiation has important therapeutic implications, as will be illustrated later in the present patient.

See box 2.

Causes of acute renal failure

Acute renal failure is a clinical term that encompasses many causes of abrupt renal impairment; that is, a fall in GFR occurring over a period of hours or days which results in impaired fluid and electrolyte homeostasis and the accumulation of nitrogenous wastes. Acute renal failure occurs in response to a wide variety of insults, the most common causes being haemody-

Table 5.2
Laboratory assessment to differentiate prerenal oliguria from established renal failure

Laboratory parameter	Prerenal	Established renal failure
Urinary [Na] (mmol/L)	< 20	> 40
Fractional Na excretion*	< 1%	> 1%
Urine:plasma osmolality ratio	> 1.5	< 1.1
Urine:plasma creatinine ratio	> 40	< 20
Plasma urea:creatinine ratio (both in mmol/L)	> 80	< 80

*Fractional excretion of Na (FE$_{Na}$)

$$= \frac{(Urine_{Na}/Plasma_{Na})}{(Urine_{Cr}/Plasma_{Cr})} \times 100\%.$$

Glomerular filtration and acute renal failure box 2

Investigations

Initial blood tests in Mrs Wood showed an elevation in the white cell count, with a neutrophilia consistent with infection. The haemoglobin was *168 g/L and haematocrit was *0.53, consistent with haemoconcentration.

The plasma urea concentration was elevated at *26 mmol/L and creatinine was elevated at *0.35 mmol/L. The plasma sodium was 145 mmol/L and the potassium was elevated at *6.1 mmol/L. Acidosis was present, indicated by the reduced bicarbonate at *18 mmol/L. The serum albumin was 48 g/L, calcium was 2.20 mmol/L and phosphate was *1.8 mmol/L.

Biochemical analysis of the urine specimen taken on admission revealed a urinary sodium concentration of 44 mmol/L and a creatinine concentration of 6.5 mmol/L. The urine osmolality was 335 mosm/kg (compare plasma of 302 mosm/kg).

From this data we can conclude that Mrs Wood's oliguria is in fact associated with acute renal failure, given the marked elevation of plasma creatinine which implies a reduced GFR. The urine parameters are suggestive of impaired renal tubular function consistent with acute tubular necrosis (ATN).

The questions now arise:

① What has caused the acute renal failure in this case?

② What is the pathology and natural history of ATN?

③ How have the plasma biochemistry abnormalities come about?

④ What complications of acute renal failure can be anticipated and treated?

(*Results outside the normal range; see Appendix.)

---

namic, immunological, toxic and obstructive. Classically, the causes of acute renal failure are divided into prerenal, renal and postrenal causes depending on the site of the initiating insult (Table 5.3).

The commonest causes of acute renal failure acquired out of hospital are prolonged ischaemic injury in some 50% of cases, and nephrotoxic injury in 35%. In hospital-acquired renal failure, the cause is usually multifactorial. The major predisposing factors include volume depletion (often caused by vomiting, diarrhoea or diuretics), and treatment with drugs

Table 5.3
Causes of acute renal failure

Prerenal	Renal	Postrenal
Hypovolaemia	Acute tubular necrosis (ischaemic or toxic)	Bilateral ureteric obstruction
Decreased effective blood volume	Interstitial nephritis	Ureteric obstruction in a single kidney
Decreased cardiac output	Glomerular disease (e.g. acute glomerulonephritis)	Bladder outflow obstruction
Renovascular obstruction	Small vessel disease (e.g. microvasculitis)	
	Intrarenal vasoconstriction (e.g. in sepsis)	
	Tubular obstruction (e.g. urate crystals)	

(such as angiotensin-converting enzyme inhibitors, angiotensin II receptor blockers or non-steroidal anti-inflammatory drugs), and radiocontrast agents. Elderly, diabetic and chronically hypertensive patients are at particular risk because of their predisposition to underlying vascular disease and poor renal autoregulatory responses. In the hospital population, hypotension, heart failure, sepsis and aminoglycoside use are common additional factors involved in the genesis of acute renal failure. Sustained circulatory failure leading to ischaemia-induced ATN accounts for the majority of cases of acute renal failure overall.

Acute tubular necrosis

When the kidney sustains a severe hypoxic insult, injury and death of tubular cells occurs, and the resulting clinicopathological syndrome is referred to as ATN. This most commonly occurs as a result of prolonged renal ischaemia during a period of hypotension. Other causes include direct toxic injury to the tubules by endogenous chemicals such as myoglobin (released from damaged muscle cells – rhabdomyolysis) or haemoglobin (released from red blood cells during acute episodes of haemolysis). Less commonly, ATN results from exposure to nephrotoxic drugs (see Chapter 11) and heavy metals.

A number of biochemical processes have been implicated in the development of injury to tubular cells, particularly following the onset of renal ischaemia. These include depletion of cellular ATP, increase in intracellular calcium, disruption of cytoskeletal structures, loss of epithelial polarity, activation of apoptosis (programmed cell death), and increased oxygen free radical production. The latter mechanism may be particularly important as a cause of tissue injury during the reperfusion phase after a period of ischaemia.

Pathology of acute tubular necrosis

Histologically, the changes in ATN are most prominent in the cells of the proximal tubule, particularly in its

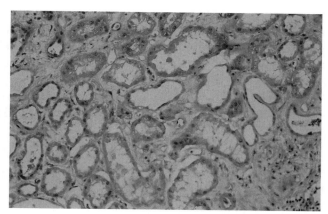

Fig. 5.7
Micrograph (stained with haematoxylin and eosin) showing acute tubular necrosis.
Note the atrophy of the tubular epithelium, the dilatation of tubules and the interstitial oedema (wide separation between adjacent tubules).

latter third (S3 segment). Blebs appear in the apical brush border, with sloughing of the brush border membrane into the lumen or involution into the cytoplasm. The integrity of the tight junctions is disrupted and loss of epithelial cell polarity occurs. Integrins, which normally contribute to cell–cell adhesion, are redistributed to the apical membrane, resulting in shedding of both live and dead cells into the lumen, which contributes to cast formation and tubular obstruction. Interstitial oedema is prominent because of leakage of tubular fluid across damaged tubular walls (Fig. 5.7). The glomeruli are generally relatively well preserved.

Pathophysiology of acute tubular necrosis

A variety of mechanisms have been proposed to explain the persistence of reduced glomerular filtration in the context of ATN, even after the instigating stimulus has been corrected or removed. These include

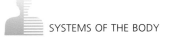
sustained renal vasoconstriction, probably mediated by intrarenal humoral factors, reduced glomerular permeability, mechanical obstruction by sloughed cells and proteinaceous casts, and back-leak of filtrate from the tubular lumen. It is likely that a different pattern of mechanisms is involved depending on the exact cause or contributing factors in a given case of ATN.

Course of acute tubular necrosis

Impaired renal function and oligoanuria during ATN typically persist for 1 week or more, after which complete cellular recovery can occur, accompanied by a return of GFR towards normal and a marked increase in urine output. This recovery is due to epithelial cell regeneration, probably under the control of locally produced peptide growth factors such as insulin-like growth factor 1 and epidermal growth factor.

As long as renal function can be temporarily replaced with a form of dialysis during the period of suppressed GFR, with correction of electrolyte disturbances and maintenance of adequate nutrition the patient can recover and reattain normal renal function. Close attention to replacement of fluid and electrolytes is important during the early recovery phase, as a period of polyuria and uncontrolled electrolyte loss is common as tubular regeneration proceeds.

See box 3.

Overview: assessment and management of a patient with acute renal failure

A logical approach to the evaluation of a patient with acute renal failure is presented in Table 5.4. All patients presenting with acute renal failure require a careful history and examination, urinalysis and urine microscopy, plasma and urine biochemistry analysis and full blood count. In general, urinary tract obstruction should be excluded early on with a renal ultrasound. Subsequent investigations depend on whether the cause of acute renal failure is considered to be caused by prerenal, renal or postrenal pathology. Clues should also be sought to determine whether there is a background of chronic renal failure, which is suggested by anaemia, hyperphosphataemia, hypocalcaemia and small kidney size.

Biochemical changes in acute renal failure

When the kidneys fail over a short time period, the metabolic disturbances which occur reflect failure of their normal homeostatic role in maintaining body

Glomerular filtration and acute renal failure box 3

Progress

Mrs Wood's acute renal failure was attributed to ATN on the basis of prolonged renal ischaemia caused by dehydration, hypotension and sepsis, on a background of treatment with a diuretic and an angiotensin-converting enzyme (ACE) inhibitor.

Initial treatment consisted of ceasing her antihypertensives, rehydration with normal saline and commencement of intravenous antibiotics (ampicillin 1 g tds, metronidazole 500 mg tds and gentamicin 240 mg in a single initial dose). A surgical opinion was sought, and a conservative approach to management of her diverticular abscess was recommended in the first instance.

Over the following 2 days, Mrs Wood's general condition improved considerably, with loss of fever and improvement of tissue hydration, with the blood pressure rising to 150/85. However, her urine output remained very poor and the plasma creatinine concentration increased further to *0.45 mmol/L. Mild hyperkalaemia and acidosis persisted.

In view of these developments, consistent with a sustained reduction in GFR due to tubular necrosis, Mrs Wood was seen by the consultant nephrologist who arranged for her to commence intermittent haemodialysis via a temporary catheter inserted into her jugular vein. She tolerated these treatments well, and there was further improvement in her clinical condition and electrolytes over the following week. She received parenteral nutrition over this period.

Ten days after admission, an increase in urine output was noted, which was then matched by an increase in her intravenous fluid therapy. Over the next few days, her plasma urea and creatinine concentrations started to fall towards normal, and her dialysis was discontinued. She was now eating and drinking, and was recommenced on an antihypertensive drug regime to control her blood pressure. On surgical review, the decision was made to defer surgery on her bowel until further settling of her inflammatory mass had occurred. She was discharged from hospital 2 weeks after admission.

fluid volume and composition within a narrow normal range. Changes in plasma biochemistry usually seen in this situation are shown in Table 5.5. It is important to note that this table does not include any direct indication of altered body fluid volume in acute renal failure. As a result of an impaired capacity to excrete

Table 5.4
Assessment of a patient with acute renal failure

Procedure	Information sought
Clinical history and examination	Clues to the cause of acute renal failure (see Table 5.3)
	Indicators of severity of metabolic disturbance
	Estimate of volume status (hydration)(see Table 2.1)
Urinalysis and urine microscopy	Markers of glomerular or tubulointerstitial inflammation, urinary tract infection or crystal uropathy
Plasma biochemistry	To assess extent of GFR reduction and metabolic consequences
Urine biochemistry	To differentiate prerenal from established renal failure (see Table 5.2)
Full blood count	To determine presence of anaemia, leucocytosis and platelet consumption
Renal ultrasound	To determine kidney size, presence of obstruction, abnormal renal parenchymal texture
Plus, where appropriate:	
Abdominal CT scan	To define structural abnormalities of the kidneys or urinary tract
Radionuclide scan	To assess abnormal renal perfusion
Cystoscopy +/– retrograde pyelograms	To evaluate/relieve urinary tract obstruction
Renal biopsy	To define pathology of renal parenchymal disease

CT, computed tomography; GFR, glomerular filtration rate.

Table 5.5
Changes in plasma biochemistry in acute renal failure

Hyperkalaemia
Decreased bicarbonate
Elevated urea
Elevated creatinine
Elevated uric acid
Hypocalcaemia
Hyperphosphataemia

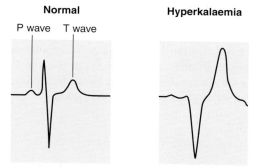

Fig. 5.8
Electrocardiogram in severe hyperkalaemia. Note the widening of the QRS complex and the high peaked T waves compared to the normal tracing. The plasma potassium in this patient was 7.6 mmol/L.

fluid, this is usually manifested as hypervolaemia and, in extreme cases, pulmonary oedema, which must be assessed clinically and radiologically.

Hyperkalaemia results from potassium retention due to a failure of filtration and tubular secretion of potassium by the damaged kidney. There is, in addition, an increased potassium load associated with some causes of acute renal failure such as muscle crush injury. This electrolyte disturbance is particularly serious because of its potential to produce life-threatening cardiac asystole through its effect on the excitability of cardiac conducting tissue. It can also lead to profound skeletal muscle weakness.

Other factors which may contribute to hyperkalaemia include conditions or drugs which directly influence the capacity of the distal tubule to secrete potassium, as is sometimes seen in cases where the urinary tract is infected and obstructed, or in low aldosterone states, or when potassium-sparing diuretics or ACE inhibitors are being used. Acidosis also contributes to hyperkalaemia by transcellular exchange of potassium ions for hydrogen ions.

ECG abnormalities are often the first indication that severe hyperkalaemia is present (Fig. 5.8). Such changes, usually associated with a serum potassium greater than 6.5 mmol/L, require emergency treatment with an infusion of calcium gluconate to stabilize the membrane potential in the cardiac conducting tissue, followed by agents to shift potassium into cells (nebulized beta-agonists, intravenous sodium bicarbonate, intravenous glucose and insulin). These measures must be accompanied by interventions to remove potassium from the body (ion exchange resins or dialysis).

Metabolic acidosis (reflected by a low bicarbonate) occurs in renal failure because of the retention of organic acids, and failure of the kidney to secrete and excrete the net hydrogen ion load (see Chapter 4). An additional acid load may be generated in some settings of acute renal failure, such as with lactate production in the presence of poor tissue perfusion.

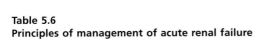

GLOMERULAR FILTRATION AND ACUTE RENAL FAILURE

Table 5.6
Principles of management of acute renal failure

Problem	Management
Fluid volume disturbance	Rehydrate if hypovolaemic; withhold fluid and give high dose diuretic if hypervolaemic; dialysis for resistant pulmonary oedema
Metabolic disturbances	
Hyperkalaemia	Intravenous calcium, bicarbonate, glucose plus insulin; oral/rectal ion exchange resin; dialysis
Acidosis	Bicarbonate supplements; dialysis
Uraemic syndrome	Dialysis
Infection	Antibiotics ± surgery if appropriate
Bleeding	dDAVP to improve platelet dysfunction; dialysis
Nutritional deficiencies	Enteral or parenteral feeding in conjunction with dialysis

dDAVP, des-amino D-arginine vasopressin, a synthetic analogue of vasopressin (the naturally occurring antidiuretic hormone) which also has the property of enhancing platelet function.

Elevated urea and creatinine are manifestations of the retention of nitrogenous products of metabolism because of reduced filtration. Both substances have additional significance as markers of the GFR, with creatinine being more useful for this purpose (see above). Clinical manifestations probably relate most to the elevation in urea, which produces the syndrome of uraemia characterized by impaired mental function (drowsiness and confusion), **anorexia,** nausea and vomiting and, in severe cases, **asterixis** and **pericarditis**.

Hyperphosphataemia also results from failure of filtration, but is aggravated in situations in which a high phosphate load is generated (such as tissue breakdown in rhabdomyolysis or **tumour lysis syndrome**). The total plasma calcium is generally low at the onset of acute renal failure, although this often normalizes or overcorrects as recovery proceeds.

Complications of acute renal failure

Complications may arise as a result of the renal failure itself or the illnesses associated with the development of renal failure.

The most important factors in contributing to morbidity and mortality rates are cardiovascular complications arising from fluid overload, arrhythmias, acute myocardial ischaemia and hypertension. Systemic infection is another major cause of adverse outcomes in acute renal failure. This is probably due to the effect of the abnormal metabolic environment on immunological functions, although it often relates directly to the cause of the acute renal failure, such as Gram-negative septicaemia or burns.

Neurological disturbances often parallel the rate of rise of blood urea, sometimes resulting in a depressed level of consciousness or seizures.

Gastrointestinal haemorrhage occurs frequently in these patients, often on the basis of an impaired coagulation mechanism. This may be caused by a platelet function defect induced by uraemia, reduced tissue integrity predisposing to bleeding, and sometimes systemic coagulopathy related to the primary cause of renal failure.

Another factor contributing to high morbidity and mortality rates in acute renal failure is impaired nutritional status. Factors contributing to this may include:

- anorexia in the period before development of renal failure
- a catabolic state commonly associated with renal failure
- uncontrolled acidosis which accelerates protein breakdown
- inadequate provision of nutrients in the early phase of management.

Management of acute renal failure

The principles of management of acute renal failure can be summarized as shown in Table 5.6. Note that the table does not include the measures required to correct the underlying cause of acute renal failure, e.g. relieving urinary tract obstruction when present.

It should be clear from the above that the availability of renal replacement therapy in the form of acute dialysis is of critical importance in saving lives from this medical emergency. This can be a particularly cost-effective form of intervention given that the kidney has the capacity for complete recovery in many of the conditions underlying this presentation.

Self-assessment case study

A previously well 32-year-old man is brought to the emergency department having been involved in a motor vehicle accident. The circumstances of the accident are initially unclear. However, the ambulance officers who attended the accident noted that he was trapped in the vehicle for 3 h before being freed. At this time he was hypotensive with a systolic blood pressure of 80 mmHg, and had significant injuries to his lower limbs with probable fracture of both femora. He was initially treated with colloid and subsequently crystalloid fluid resuscitation, and his systolic blood pressure stabilized at 100 mmHg. At the time of admission to the emergency department, abdominal, thoracic and cerebral injuries were excluded and his injuries were assessed as being confined to his lower limbs. He was tachycardic and his blood pressure was 100/60 mmHg, and his jugular venous pressure was not visible even though he was lying flat. In preparation for surgical stabilization of his lower limbs, he had a urinary catheter inserted and 50 ml of dark urine which tested strongly positive for blood on urinalysis was drained, after which minimal urine output was documented.

Initial laboratory investigations revealed the following results:

*Haemoglobin 79 g/L
Sodium 140 mmol/L
*Potassium 7.8 mmol/L
Chloride 98 mmol/L
*Bicarbonate 11 mmol/L

*Urea 13 mmol/L
*Creatinine 0.19 mmol/L.
(*Results outside normal range; see Appendix.)

After studying this chapter you should be able to answer the following questions:

① What are the factors involved in the development of this man's acute renal failure?

② What additional biochemical abnormalities are likely to be present?

③ Describe the immediate treatment of his acute renal failure.

④ Describe in general terms the expected course and prognosis of his renal failure.

Answers see page 147

Self-assessment questions

① Describe the factors involved in determining glomerular filtration.

② Define the renal clearance of a substance and explain why clearance of creatinine reflects kidney function.

③ What are the clinical and laboratory features that differentiate physiological oliguria from acute tubular necrosis?

Answers see page 147

PROTEINURIA AND THE NEPHROTIC SYNDROME

6

Chapter objectives

After studying this chapter you should be able to:

① Describe the anatomy of the normal glomerulus, including its three cell types and their arrangement, and the structure of the glomerular capillary wall and glomerular basement membrane (GBM).

② Discuss the components of normal and abnormal proteinuria, and differentiate tubular and glomerular proteinuria.

③ Understand the role of the glomerulus and its components (cells and GBM) in preventing proteinuria.

④ Discuss the pathophysiology and differential diagnosis of oedema.

⑤ Understand the features and pathophysiology of nephrotic syndrome and its complications.

⑥ List the main diseases that cause nephrotic syndrome in children and adults.

⑦ Describe the renal histopathological features of minimal change disease.

⑧ Discuss the natural history of minimal change disease, and the other major causes of nephrotic syndrome.

⑨ Discuss the response to treatment of the major causes of nephrotic syndrome.

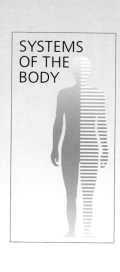

SYSTEMS OF THE BODY

Introduction

To produce an ultrafiltrate of plasma as the first stage in urine production, the glomerulus must retain plasma proteins within the lumen of its capillary network. This ability to retain plasma proteins by preventing their filtration into the tubular lumen is determined by the size- and charge-selective properties of the glomerular capillary wall (GCW). When diseases damage the integrity of this wall, plasma proteins may escape across it into the tubular lumen.

The proximal segments of the nephron have the capacity to reabsorb and metabolize very efficiently any proteins that appear in the tubular lumen. Under normal circumstances, small plasma proteins which are able to pass across the GCW are taken up (endocytosed) by proximal tubular cells, where they are broken down in lysosomes. However, protein may appear in the final urine (proteinuria) if the amount filtered by the glomerulus overwhelms tubular reabsorptive mechanisms, or if tubular cells are damaged.

Severe proteinuria may damage the kidney, or have systemic consequences because of loss of albumin and other proteins from the blood.

In this chapter, the causes and consequences of proteinuria will be considered and illustrated by a case of severe proteinuria occurring in a child.

See box 1.

Pathophysiology of oedema formation

Oedema literally means 'swelling', and refers to the accumulation of fluid within the tissues. This fluid is located outside the vascular system in the interstitial space (see Chapter 2).

Under normal circumstances, the balance between hydrostatic and osmotic pressure gradients (Starling's forces) across capillary walls prevents oedema formation (Fig. 6.1A). The hydrostatic pressure of the column of blood within systemic capillaries is determined by the pumping action of the heart and resistance to flow within the arterial tree, and capacitance of the venous system. Capillary hydrostatic pressure varies in different tissues, but is on average about 25 mmHg. This favours the movement of plasma filtrate into the surrounding interstitial compartment, which has a lower hydrostatic pressure. This hydrostatic pressure gradient is opposed by osmotic forces which favour the movement of fluid from the interstitium (which has a colloid osmotic pressure, or oncotic pressure, of about 1 mmHg) into the capillary lumen (where plasma proteins exert an oncotic pressure of about 25 mmHg). In fact, capillary hydrostatic pressure falls along the length of the capillary, whereas capillary oncotic pressure rises as water moves into the interstitial space.

Proteinuria and the nephrotic syndrome box 1

Generalized oedema

Kylie Major presented to her general practitioner (GP) with facial swelling of 3 days duration. Kylie was a 6-year-old girl who had been completely healthy in the past and had had no antecedent illnesses before presentation. Her GP found obvious pitting oedema (swelling which can be indented by digital compression) in her face and around her ankles. Her blood pressure was 95/60. Her jugular venous pressure was normal, her chest was clear to **auscultation** and there was no shifting dullness on percussion of her abdomen, indicating that there was no clinically obvious ascites (free peritoneal fluid). Dipstick analysis of a fresh urine sample was strongly positive for protein but negative for blood. Her GP thought her generalized oedema was most likely caused by proteinuria.

Consideration of the presenting features of this patient leads to the following questions:

① What are the forces which prevent the development of oedema normally?

② What are the major diseases that cause oedema? How are the forces opposing oedema formation disrupted in these conditions?

③ How does proteinuria cause oedema?

These questions will be addressed in the first section of this chapter.

Thus these forces favour net water movement into the interstitium at the arterial end of the capillary (hydrostatic > oncotic pressure), balanced under normal conditions by an equivalent movement of water in the other direction at the venous end (oncotic > hydrostatic pressure). Oedema fluid within the interstitial space is limited also by drainage via lymphatic vessels.

The above principles apply to other capillary beds, but the details of the forces involved vary (see, for example, Chapter 5 for a discussion of forces in the glomerulus, a capillary bed designed to achieve net movement of fluid out of the lumen).

Oedema arises because of a localized or generalized disruption of Starling's forces within capillaries, or because of a failure of lymphatic drainage of the interstitial space (Fig. 6.1B). Thus, factors which favour oedema formation include a loss of integrity of the capillary wall, an increase in hydrostatic pressure within the capillary lumen (e.g. caused by high venous pressures within the systemic or pulmonary circula-

A Starting's forces acting across systemic capillary walls

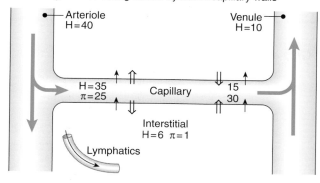

B Factors favouring oedema formation

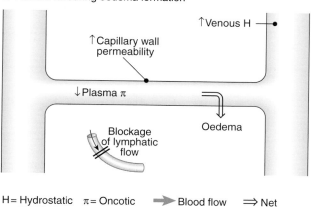

H = Hydrostatic π = Oncotic   → Blood flow   ⇒ Net
pressure   pressure   → Direction   movement
in mmHg   in mmHg   of force   of fluid

Fig. 6.1

(A) Starling's forces acting across systemic capillary walls. The net movement of fluid depends on the balance between capillary and interstitial hydrostatic (H) and oncotic (π) pressures. Representative values (in mmHg) are shown. (B) Factors favouring oedema formation. Reduction in plasma oncotic pressure, increase in capillary wall permeability or venous hydrostatic pressure, or lymphatic blockage will increase oedema formation.

tion as occurs in congestive cardiac failure, and within portal veins in **cirrhosis**), reduction in plasma oncotic pressure due to hypoalbuminaemia, or obstruction of lymphatic flow. The main causes of oedema are listed in Table 6.1.

If oedema formation were determined only by Starling's forces in capillaries, then body weight should not increase. However, in most conditions causing generalized oedema (Table 6.1), the kidneys actively retain salt and water, causing weight gain and aggravating the build-up of oedema fluid. Salt and water retention in these circumstances may arise as a response to a reduction in 'effective' arterial blood

volume, leading to a number of responses designed to protect against hypovolaemia (see Chapter 2). These responses include systemic haemodynamic changes which occur quickly, and intrarenal changes which lead to salt and water retention over days to weeks. The intrarenal factors include:

- reflex activation of the sympathetic nervous system
- activation of the renin–angiotensin–aldosterone system and vasopressin release
- resistance to the action of natriuretic peptides
- altered glomerular haemodynamics
- peritubular forces in the proximal tubule.

These neuronal, hormonal and intrarenal mechanisms, which together augment sodium reabsorption at multiple sites along the nephron, are discussed in more detail in Chapter 2.

The predominant site of oedema can give a clue to the aetiology. Thus, with right-sided heart failure, peripheral oedema (affecting the extremities) should be accompanied by a raised jugular venous pressure and hepatic congestion. With left-sided heart failure, pulmonary congestion alone is expected. With cirrhosis, ascites (fluid accumulation in the peritoneal cavity) is seen earlier than in other causes of generalized oedema because of portal venous hypertension. Peripheral oedema also occurs with cirrhosis owing to hypoalbuminaemia.

When there is marked proteinuria, peripheral and/or facial oedema (Fig. 6.2A) develops because of hypoalbuminaemia. This combination of findings is called the nephrotic syndrome (or nephrosis). The site of oedema is also influenced by the effect of gravity. Thus, in ambulant patients, mild oedema is frequently seen first around the ankles (where venous hydrostatic pressure is highest in the erect posture), whereas in bedridden patients it may be over the sacrum as this is the most dependent position. With severe nephrotic syndrome, oedema can be more widespread and may involve the lungs and pleural and peritoneal cavities (Fig. 6.2B). If renal salt and water retention is a predominant pathophysiological event, as occurs in some forms of nephrosis (particularly where the glomerular filtration rate (GFR) is reduced), the blood volume may be increased and jugular venous pressure raised.

The three main generalized oedema states are congestive cardiac failure, cirrhosis and nephrotic syndrome. These may be differentiated by the finding of signs of cardiac disease in the case of congestive cardiac failure, of liver failure in the case of cirrhosis, and of heavy proteinuria in cases of nephrotic syndrome. The latter is clearly the problem in the present patient and will be the subject of the rest of this chapter.

Table 6.1
Main causes of oedema

	Pathophysiological factors	Predominant site
Local		
Infection, trauma	Capillary leak	Local
Venous obstruction (e.g. thrombosis)	Increased venous hydrostatic pressure	Local
Lymphatic obstruction	Lymphatic obstruction	Local
Generalized		
Congestive cardiac failure	Increased venous hydrostatic pressure, renal salt and water retention	Jugular veins (intravascular, not 'oedema'), lower limb, pulmonary
Cirrhosis	Decreased plasma oncotic pressure, renal salt and water retention, increased venous hydrostatic pressure	Ascites, lower limb
Nephrotic syndrome	Decreased plasma oncotic pressure, renal salt and water retention	Facial, lower limb
Septicaemia	Capillary leak	Lower limb, pulmonary
Allergic reactions (angio-oedema)	Capillary leak	Facial
Cyclical ('idiopathic')	?	Lower limb
Drugs	Increased venous hydrostatic pressure, renal salt and water retention	Lower limb

Glomerular anatomy and the filtration barrier

Each human kidney contains about one million glomeruli, each of which is a specialized capillary network fed by a single afferent arteriole and drained by a single efferent arteriole. The glomerulus is populated by three intrinsic cells: the capillary endothelial cell, the epithelial cell which lies over it with the glomerular basement membrane (GBM) in between, and the mesangial cell. Under normal circumstances, protein is largely excluded from glomerular filtrate by an intact GCW. As shown in Fig. 6.3, the GCW comprises three layers: the endothelial cell, the GBM and the visceral glomerular epithelial cell (GEC). Each layer appears to act as a barrier to filtration of protein, but this function is subserved predominantly by the GBM and by the slit pore between cytoplasmic extensions ('foot processes' or 'podocytes') of the GEC. The visceral GEC can be visualized as a small-headed octopus with its many discrete feet (podocytes) draped over and covering the outer surface of each glomerular loop. Between the podocytes are slit pores, across which are spread thin diaphragms consisting of newly recognized proteins such as nephrin.

The GBM also consists of specialized structural proteins, including certain collagens and charged heparin-like molecules. These molecules are arranged so that discrete pores prevent movement of large molecules (size selectivity) and charged ions (charge selectivity) across the GBM. Thus albumin, which is negatively charged and has a molecular weight of 67 000 D, does not pass across the normal GBM. Haemoglobin has a similar molecular weight to albumin but is not charged; therefore when it is released from red blood cells (haemolysis), it can pass across the GBM and is excreted in the urine (haemoglobinuria). Smaller proteins such as myoglobin (17 000 D) and monomeric light chains (22 000 D) pass across freely, whereas larger molecules such as ferritin (480 000 D) may only pass across severely disrupted GBMs.

Although the mesangial cell is not anatomically part of the GCW, it can alter the filtration of proteins because of its contractile properties (which alter the surface area of GCW available for filtration) and its ability to absorb, metabolize and discharge macromolecules into renal lymphatic channels.

Normal and abnormal proteinuria

Normal urine contains a small amount of protein, less than 150 mg/day in adults. Normal urinary protein consists of proteins of small molecular weight which have been filtered across the GCW and not reabsorbed by tubular cells, and proteins such as Tamm–Horsfall protein which are secreted by tubular cells. Heavy exercise, fever and prolonged standing ('orthostasis') may increase proteinuria in otherwise normal individuals. As explained above, larger proteins such as albumin are found in only very small amounts in normal urine.

Abnormal proteinuria may arise because of failure of the GCW filtration barrier ('glomerular proteinuria') or decreased protein reabsorption into, or increased protein release from, tubular epithelial cells ('tubular proteinuria'; see Fig. 6.4). Tubular proteinuria consists of low molecular weight proteins (generally less than 40 000 D) and usually amounts to less than 1 g/day. Glomerular proteinuria consists of proteins of greater

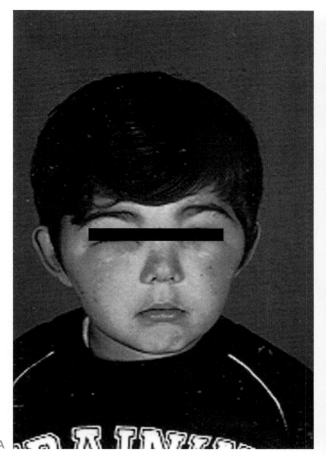
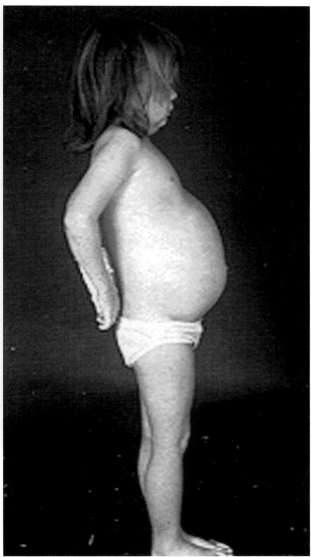

Fig. 6.2
Patients with severe nephrotic syndrome, showing (A) facial oedema and (B) ascites.

molecular size and may be up to many grams per day. In some glomerular diseases in which the injury is of a limited nature, such as minimal change disease, proteins much larger than albumin may be excluded from the urine ('selective proteinuria'), whereas with more extensive damage immunoglobulins and even larger proteins may be found in the urine ('non-selective proteinuria'). When glomerular proteinuria is severe, nephrotic syndrome may develop, as occurred with the current patient.

The principal causes of proteinuria are listed in Table 6.2. The most important of these in clinical terms are those conditions which cause damage to the glomerulus. Glomerular disease may be primary (glomerulonephritis) or secondary to systemic diseases such as

diabetes mellitus. In addition, glomerular disease may occur as a component or consequence of widespread renal scarring which occurs late in the course of any chronic renal disease. In the latter situation the glomerular scarring is called 'glomerulosclerosis'.

See box 2.

Nephrotic syndrome

Clinical features

Nephrotic syndrome (or nephrosis) consists of a diagnostic triad of heavy proteinuria, which leads to hypoalbuminaemia, which in turn causes oedema (Table 6.3).

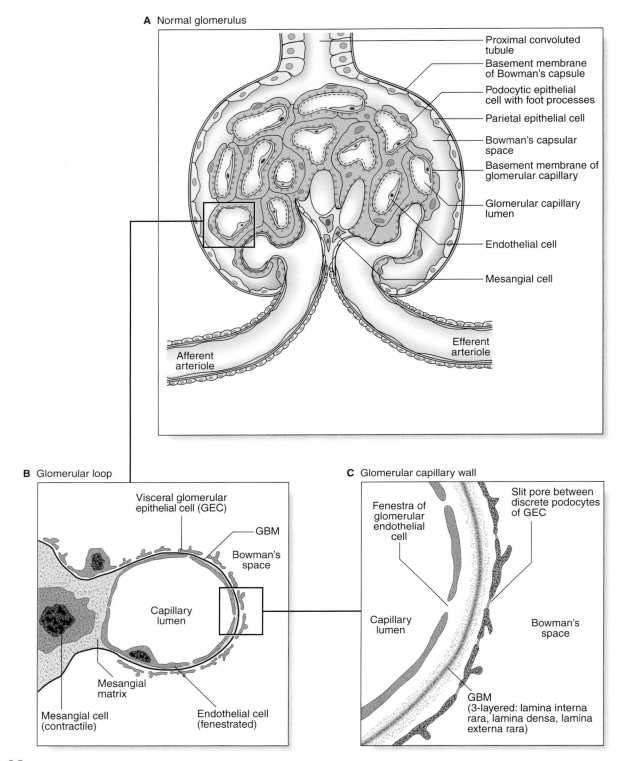

Fig. 6.3
(A) Structure of the normal glomerulus, which is a capillary network fed by an afferent arteriole, and drained by an efferent arteriole; (B) glomerular loop, consisting of a capillary lumen lying beneath glomerular epithelial cells (GEC) and adjacent to mesangium; (C) glomerular capillary wall, comprising glomerular endothelial cells surrounded by the glomerular basement membrane (GBM) and GEC.

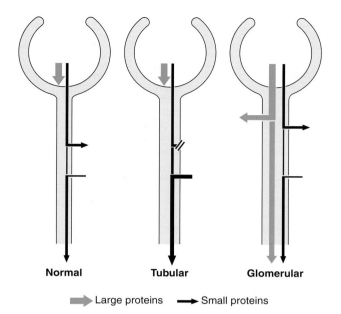

Large proteins → **Small proteins**

Fig. 6.4
Proteinuria, occurring in normal kidneys or as a result of tubular or glomerular disease.

Table 6.2
Principal causes of proteinuria

Normal kidneys
    Normal (< 150 mg/24 h)
    Exercise
    Fever
    Orthostasis
Abnormal kidneys
    Tubular diseases (≤ 1 g/24 h)
    Glomerular disease (> 1 or 2 g/24 h)
        Primary glomerulonephritis
        Secondary glomerular disease in:
            systemic diseases such as diabetes mellitus, **amyloidosis**
            generalized renal scarring

Proteinuria and the nephrotic syndrome box 2

Investigations

Kylie's GP organized some blood and urine tests. Her serum creatinine was normal, and serum albumin was very low at *13 g/L. Microscopic examination of spun urinary sediment was normal except for the presence of many hyaline (proteinaceous) casts. Urinary protein excretion was *6 g/day, and consisted mainly of albumin. Serum cholesterol was *9.6 mmol/L and serum triglycerides were normal.

When Kylie returned to be reviewed by her GP 2 days later, she had gained an extra 3 kg in weight and her oedema was worse. In addition, she was complaining of pain in her right calf, which appeared to be more swollen than the left. Her GP suspected a deep vein thrombosis in her right calf and treated her with anticoagulants.

In summary, the results of Kylie's tests indicated that her generalized oedema was caused by hypoalbuminaemia, which in turn was due to heavy proteinuria. As the proteinuria was predominantly albuminuria, it can be considered as 'selective', suggesting a restricted injury to the glomerular filtration barrier.

Her subsequent clinical course raises the following questions:

① Why did the oedema progress?

② Was the hypercholesterolaemia related to her renal disease?

③ What was the relationship between her renal disease and the deep venous thrombosis?

(Values outside normal range; see Appendix.)

Complications of nephrotic syndrome are relatively common, and their frequency increases with the severity of the proteinuria. Some of the complications arise because of loss of 'protective' factors in the urine, and others are caused by increased hepatic production of 'damaging' factors, apparently as part of a generalized compensatory hepatic synthetic response primarily involving albumin. The major complications of nephrosis and their pathogenesis are described in Table 6.3. These complications are clinically relevant and, in untreated nephrosis, have an important bearing on what happens to the patient.

It has been established that this patient has severe nephrotic syndrome with complications. The next questions to be asked include the following.

- What type of kidney disease caused the nephrosis?
- Can and should the disease be treated?

These questions will be answered below.
See box 3.

Renal biopsy

Percutaneous renal biopsy, in which a small specimen of kidney tissue is obtained under local anaesthesia using a specialized needle, can be used to establish diagnosis and prognosis in patients with suspected renal parenchymal disease, including those with nephrotic syndrome. Although it is a safe procedure,

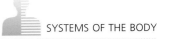

Proteinuria and the nephrotic syndrome box 3

Diagnosis

Kylie was referred to a nephrologist to have a renal biopsy. However, the nephrologist informed Kylie's GP that in this particular instance there was no need to perform a renal biopsy as the clinical features and (subsequent) response to treatment predicted both diagnosis and prognosis with high sensitivity and specificity.

This portion of the patient's history raises the following questions:

① How can the glomerular disease be diagnosed?

② Is a kidney biopsy always necessary to make the diagnosis?

Table 6.3
Nephrotic syndrome

	Pathophysiology
Diagnostic triad	
Proteinuria > 3.5 g/day	Disease of glomerular capillary wall
Serum albumin < 30 g/L	Urinary protein loss
Oedema	Low plasma oncotic pressure
	Salt and water retention by kidneys
Complications	
Hypercholesterolaemia	Increased hepatic synthesis and reduced metabolism of lipoproteins
Thrombosis	Venous obstruction caused by oedema
	Increased hepatic synthesis of clotting factors
	Urinary loss of antithrombotic proteins
Infection	Urinary loss of immunoglobulins and other defence proteins
Renal failure	Intravascular volume depletion (acute)
	Intrarenal oedema (acute)
	Primary renal disease causing glomerular damage
	Proteinuria causing interstitial inflammation
Malnutrition	Severe protein loss

it can be complicated by bleeding and so is used selectively. It may not be used when the diagnosis is in little doubt, when it is unlikely to lead to a change in therapy, or when the chance of complication is greater than usual.

Renal biopsy specimens are examined by light microscopy with standard and special stains, by electron microscopy and by immunofluorescence

Table 6.4
Renal biopsy: parameters

Light microscopy	
Glomerulus	Glomerular capillary wall thickness, cellularity, matrix, sclerosis
	Focal *versus* diffuse, segmental *versus* global
Blood vessels	Wall thickness, inflammation, occlusion
Tubule cells	Hypertrophy, atrophy
Interstitium	Inflammation, fibrosis
Electron microscopy	
Glomerular epithelial cell podocytes: discrete *versus* fused	
Glomerular basement membrane: thickness, regularity	
Site of electron-dense deposits: mesangial, subendothelial, subepithelial	
Immunofluorescence microscopy	
Glomerular pattern	Capillary wall *versus* mesangial, linear *versus* granular
Ligand of fluorescent antibody	Immunoglobulins, complement component, light chain

microscopy. The main parameters examined are listed in Table 6.4. Abnormalities may be segmental (involving part of a glomerulus only) or global (the whole glomerulus), and focal (involving a few glomeruli only) or diffuse (most glomeruli).

The classification of glomerular disease depends largely on histopathological features of renal biopsy specimens. There are many types of glomerular disease, and the classification system is somewhat complicated and is revised every few years or so. Therefore, the student should not aim to become an expert. A basic understanding of how renal biopsies are examined and of a few important varieties of glomerular disease (described below and in Chapters 7 and 8) is sufficient for most non-nephrologists.

With minimal change disease, light and immunofluorescence microscopy are normal. The only abnormality is diffuse fusion of podocytes of the GEC seen on electron microscopy (Fig. 6.5).

Causes of nephrotic syndrome

The main causes of nephrotic syndrome are listed in Table 6.5. The condition may arise as an isolated (primary) pathology, or as a component of a systemic disease.

In a child with new onset nephrotic syndrome and normal blood pressure, benign (or inactive) urinary sediment (see Chapter 7) and normal serum creatinine, minimal change disease is by far the most likely diagnosis. The patient's age and associated clinical features are very useful in predicting the diagnosis in other

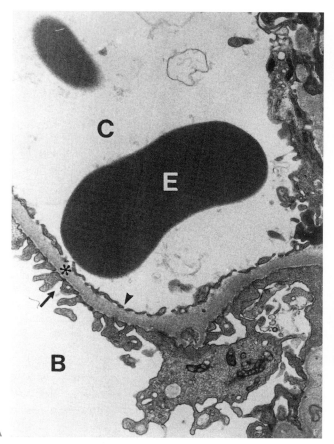
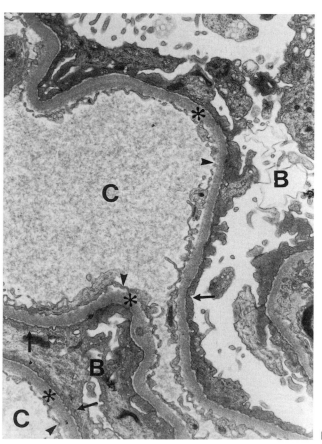

A

B

Fig. 6.5

Electron micrograph of (A) normal glomerular capillary wall (GCW) and (B) GCW from a patient with minimal change disease showing extensive fusion of the foot processes (podocytes) of glomerular epithelial cells. C, capillary lumen; B, Bowman's space; *, basement membrane; arrow head, fenestrated glomerular endothelial cell; arrow, podocytes (which are normally discrete, but fused in minimal change disease); E, red blood cell.

Table 6.5
Major causes of nephrotic syndrome

	Usual age	Response to treatment	Risk of chronic renal failure
Primary			
Minimal change disease	Child or adolescent	Yes	No
Focal sclerosing GN	Child or adolescent, adult, elderly	(Yes)	Yes
Membranous GN	Adult, elderly	(Yes)	Yes
Mesangiocapillary GN	Adult	Yes	Yes
Secondary			
Diabetic nephropathy	Adult, elderly	(No)	Yes
Amyloidosis	(Adult)*, elderly	(No)	Yes
Systemic lupus erythematosus	Adult, elderly	Yes	Yes

*Less frequent. Other parentheses indicate that this is sometimes the case. GN, glomerulonephritis.

cases, though a renal biopsy would usually be performed. Membranous glomerulonephritis is the principal cause of nephrotic syndrome in adults. It usually occurs in isolation ('primary' or 'idiopathic'), but sometimes develops as a complication of diseases such as **systemic lupus erythematosus** or cancer. Focal sclerosing glomerulonephritis can occur in any age group.

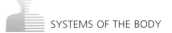
Proteinuria and the nephrotic syndrome box 4

Treatment

Kylie was treated with corticosteroids and within a few weeks her nephrotic syndrome resolved completely. Two years later her disease relapsed, and once again she responded rapidly to corticosteroids. She has remained completely well since.

Natural history and response to treatment

Treatment of nephrotic syndrome depends on the exact pathological diagnosis. In general, primary forms of glomerulonephritis causing nephrotic syndrome are treated with corticosteroids. These have an anti-inflammatory action involving depletion of T lymphocytes and impairment of polymorphonuclear leucocyte function. In some cases, immunosuppressive drugs such as cyclophosphamide are used. With secondary glomerulonephritis, treatment is directed towards the primary disease, though this may be modified considerably with renal involvement.

Response to treatment varies considerably depending on the diagnosis, as summarized in Table 6.5. Response is excellent with minimal change disease, but relapses are not infrequent. Response is much less predictable with other diagnoses. In the face of continuing nephrosis, the patient is at risk of developing complications (see Table 6.3), some of which can be prevented or treated.

Without successful treatment, nephrotic syndrome will persist in most patients, with the attendant risk of complications. Only in minimal change disease is there no risk of developing chronic renal failure.

Self-assessment case study

Eric Daniels, a 65-year-old man who had been in good health previously, presented with a 4-month history of progressive swelling of his ankles. He had no previous history of cardiac or hepatic disease, and on examination there was no evidence of cardiac or hepatic failure. Urinalysis was positive for protein (+++) but was otherwise normal.

After studying this chapter you should be able to answer the following questions:

① What is the most likely clinical diagnosis?

② Name two other features required to make this clinical diagnosis.

③ Why has the patient developed oedema?

④ List three possible complications of this condition and the pathophysiological factors involved.

⑤ In a patient of this age, what is the most likely renal histopathological diagnosis?

⑥ Describe the likely renal histopathological features.

Answers see page 148

Self-assessment questions

① List four factors which will favour the formation of oedema at the level of a capillary.

② Which three structures comprise the glomerular capillary wall?

③ What is the definition of nephrotic syndrome?

④ List the principal complications of nephrotic syndrome and their pathophysiology.

⑤ What pathological features are expected in the renal biopsy of a patient with minimal change disease?

Answers see page 148

GLOMERULO-NEPHRITIS AND THE ACUTE NEPHRITIC SYNDROME

7

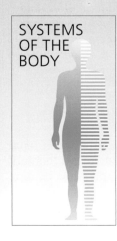

SYSTEMS
OF THE
BODY

Chapter objectives

After studying this chapter you should be able to:

① Describe the components of the acute nephritic syndrome and its variations.

② Describe other forms of presentation of glomerulonephritis (GN).

③ Understand the pathogenesis of post-streptococcal GN.

④ Differentiate acute nephritis occurring with post-streptococcal GN, IgA disease and systemic diseases.

⑤ Discuss the consequences of glomerular disease.

⑥ Describe the parameters of urinary sediment examination.

⑦ Discuss the natural history of post-streptococcal GN.

Introduction

Acute glomerulonephritis (GN) refers generally to inflammatory renal diseases affecting the glomeruli of some or all of the million nephrons of each kidney. Although this classification is based largely on the pathological appearance of glomeruli, other components of the nephron, blood vessels and renal interstitium are involved to a variable extent. Many of the acute glomerulonephritides are primary or idiopathic, whereas with others a secondary cause is identified. The pathogenesis of GN varies with the diagnosis and may involve multiple factors. With many forms it is only partially understood. In this chapter, the pathogenesis of GN will be explained by a discussion of the presentation and diagnosis of a case of acute nephritic syndrome.

There are a bewildering number of types of primary and secondary GN, and the systems of classification are overlapping and confusing. For this reason, the student is urged to concentrate only on the common or classic forms of disease which are discussed in this chapter.

See box 1.

Urinary sediment examination

To confirm the presence of renal inflammation, sediment examination should be performed on a centrifuged sample of fresh urine. Every medical student and graduate should be confident in examining urinary sediment. To allow quantification of the urinary abnormalities, this should be done in a standardized fashion. Ten millilitres of urine is spun at $2500\,g$ for $5\,min$, $9.5\,mL$ of the urine is then discarded, the sediment is resuspended in the remaining $0.5\,mL$ of urine by gentle tapping of the test tube, and this resuspended sediment is examined using a counting chamber. Normal urine may contain up to 500 red blood cells, 2000 white blood cells and 15 hyaline (but not granular or cellular) casts per millilitre.

The finding of an excess number of red or white cells may be explained by abnormalities anywhere in the urinary tract. It should be noted that a positive dipstick test for blood indicates the presence of haem pigment, whereas microscopy is required to confirm the presence of red blood cells (this is discussed in more detail in Chapter 10). When cells or cellular debris aggregate in the tubular lumen, they may form casts of the tubule. Granular or cellular (epithelial, red or white cell) casts indicate the presence of renal parenchymal disease, whereas hyaline (proteinaceous) casts are found with proteinuria. An 'active'

Glomerulonephritis and the acute nephritic syndrome box 1

Nephritic syndrome

Michael Willandra is a 22-year-old Australian aboriginal who presented to the local hospital of a western New South Wales town complaining of headache and dark urine. He had also noticed a reduction in urine output (oliguria) even though he had a normal fluid intake. In the past Michael had had frequent sore throats and skin infections. Approximately 2 weeks before presentation he had had another sore throat which resolved spontaneously after 8 days. The resident doctor noted that he had facial swelling and a blood pressure of 165/105. His jugular venous pressure was raised 2 cm and rales (sounds produced by passage of air through fluid in the lower respiratory tract) were heard on auscultation at the bases of both lungs. There was a creamy exudate on his tonsils and mild pharyngeal erythema. Dipstick analysis of urine revealed blood +++ and protein +. The doctor suspected that Michael had acute GN.

The important clinical features in this patient include the occurrence of oliguria, dark urine, hypertension and fluid overload 2 weeks after a sore throat. The questions that arise from this clinical history include the following:

① What is the pathophysiology of each of the clinical features?

② Are the clinical features interrelated?

③ What is the relationship of the sore throat to the acute illness which followed 2 weeks later?

④ What made the doctor suspect a diagnosis of GN?

The answers to these questions will be revealed in the initial sections of this chapter. Before this, however, we must discuss the examination of urinary sediment, the first and one of the most important tests in a suspected case of renal disease, which provides a non-invasive glimpse of the inflammatory processes which occur within the kidney.

sediment contains elements consistent with renal inflammation and/or cell necrosis, whereas a 'benign' sediment may contain a few cells and only hyaline casts. Fresh urine should be examined as casts may break down within 1–2 h. Figure 7.1 shows examples of urinary casts.

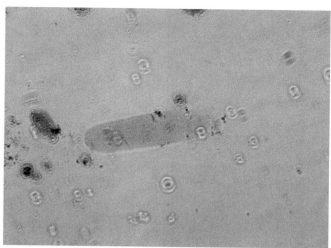
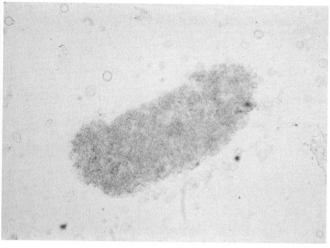

A   B

Fig. 7.1

Urinary casts: (A) hyaline, (B) red cell. Casts form within the tubular lumen and therefore take on the shape of the lumen with parallel sides. Photographs by courtesy of Prof. J. Lawrence.

Glomerulonephritis and the acute nephritic syndrome box 2

Initial investigations

Urinary sediment examination showed more than *100 red cells per microlitre, as well as a moderate number of white cell and red cell casts. Serum creatinine was elevated at *0.16 mmol/L. Based on this the doctor told Michael he had 'nephritis'.

The obvious question to be asked at this stage is: which of the clinical and laboratory features of the patient are diagnostic, characteristic or consistent with the nephritic syndrome (or nephritis)?

(*Values outside the normal range; see Appendix.)

Table 7.1
Presentation of glomerular disease

Nephritic syndrome*
Nephrotic syndrome[†]
Asymptomatic proteinuria and/or microscopic haematuria
Macroscopic haematuria
Acute renal failure
Chronic renal failure
Hypertension

*Haematuria, hypertension, renal functional impairment and oliguria. [†]Heavy proteinuria, hypoalbuminaemia and oedema.

Presentation and consequences of glomerular disease

Patients with glomerular disease may present in a number of different ways; these are listed in Table 7.1. The spectrum of presentation includes asymptomatic microscopic haematuria and/or proteinuria discovered on routine medical check, acute or chronic renal failure, hypertension, or full blown (or a limited form of) nephrotic or nephritic syndromes. The nephrotic syndrome is described in Chapter 6.

The nephritic syndrome consists of haematuria, hypertension and renal functional impairment (reduced glomerular filtration rate (GFR), reflected by the raised serum creatinine), as was found in the present case. The haematuria and active urinary sediment are indicative of renal inflammation; oliguria and renal functional impairment are a consequence of glomerular infiltration with inflammatory cells and release of vasoactive hormones and cytokines; and hypertension is the result of salt and water retention and vasoactive hormone release.

The consequences of glomerular disease and the underlying pathophysiology of each feature are described in Table 7.2. Renal functional impairment in glomerular disease is multifactorial and arises because of the acute inflammatory process (proliferation of intrinsic glomerular cells, glomerular infiltration with leucocytes and haemodynamic changes induced by vasoactive hormones and cytokines) and chronic renal scarring (caused by continuing inflammation, hypertension, proteinuria and other factors). Hypertension occurs in acute nephritis because of salt and water retention (a consequence of the reduction of GFR), glomerular capillary and arteriolar scarring, and neurohumoral changes, in particular activation of the renin–angiotensin system.

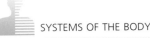

GLOMERULONEPHRITIS AND THE ACUTE NEPHRITIC SYNDROME

7

Table 7.2
Consequences of glomerular disease

Feature	Pathophysiology
Proteinuria	Impaired filtration barrier function of GCW
Haematuria	Leak into Bowman's space across GCW or into tubular lumen
Renal impairment	Structural and/or functional damage to glomeruli and tubulointerstitium
Hypertension	Salt and water retention, activation of the renin–angiotensin system

GCW, glomerular capillary wall.

Table 7.3
Important diagnostic serological tests for glomerulonephritis

Test	Diagnosis
Serum complement	
Low C3	Post-streptococcal GN, mesangiocapillary GN
Low C3 and C4	Systemic lupus erythematosus
Others	
ANA, anti-double-stranded DNA antibody	Systemic lupus erythematosus
ANCA	Microscopic polyangiitis or Wegener's granulomatosis
Anti-GBM antibody	Goodpasture's syndrome
ASOT	Post-streptococcal GN
HBsAg	Hepatitis B
Anti-HCV	Hepatitis C
HIV	AIDS
VDRL	Syphilis

ANA, antinuclear antibody; ANCA, antineutrophil cytoplasmic antibody; ASOT, antistreptococcal O titre; GBM, glomerular basement membrane; HBsAg, hepatitis B surface antigen; HCV, hepatitis C virus; VDRL, Venereal Disease Research Laboratory (serological test for syphilis).

The diagnosis of glomerular disease and, specifically, the nephritic syndrome can almost always be established by a combination of clinical features, serological tests and renal biopsy. This was the case with the current patient. These clinical and laboratory features also give clues to the pathogenesis of the disease and its complications.

See box 3.

Investigation of glomerulonephritis

There are a number of serological tests which are useful for establishing, confirming or supporting a specific diagnosis in patients with GN (Table 7.3). A positive test result suggests the primary diagnosis but does not prove that it is the cause of the renal disease. Some of these serological abnormalities are actually involved in the pathogenesis of the renal lesion, and will be discussed in more detail later in this chapter.

Renal biopsy usually establishes the diagnosis definitively. The components of renal biopsy examination are discussed in Chapter 6 (see Table 6.4). In the current patient the history, positive ASOT, low serum C3 and renal biopsy appearances were all consistent with a diagnosis of post-streptococcal GN.

Differential diagnosis of acute glomerulonephritis

GN may occur in isolation or as part of a multisystem disease. Amongst diseases in which GN is the sole manifestation, a specific precipitant is recognized in only a few. In the current case, the precipitant was a streptococcal throat infection occurring 2 weeks before the onset of GN. This once common disease is seen less frequently nowadays, except in underprivileged populations. The streptococcal infection may also be a skin infection. A similar type of GN can been seen following bacterial infections of other types (postinfectious GN).

Many patients presenting with other types of GN give a history of a respiratory illness in the preceding days to weeks. Only in some patients is the respiratory illness of definite pathogenetic significance. A common form of GN that needs to be distinguished from post-streptococcal GN is IgA disease (or mesangial IgA nephropathy). IgA disease is a common type of GN, characterized by acute nephritis and, in particular, macroscopic haematuria occurring at the time or within a few days of a viral sore throat. The shorter prodrome and its frequently recurrent nature help to distinguish it at presentation from poststreptococcal GN (Table 7.4 and Fig. 7.3).

Acute nephritic syndrome can occur in a number of conditions that are either restricted to the kidney or involve multiple organs (systemic diseases). Some of the important examples are listed in Table 7.5. Amongst these, IgA disease is the only common disease. Nevertheless, it is important to consider the other conditions because, without rapid treatment, irreversible renal failure may develop. Rapidly progressive GN, in which renal failure develops over a period of days to weeks, is characteristic of several of these conditions, including primary crescentic GN, microscopic polyangiitis and Goodpasture's syndrome.

Pathogenesis of acute glomerulonephritis

Current classification systems for GN are confusing, which is not surprising given the incomplete know-

Glomerulonephritis and the acute nephritic syndrome box 3

Diagnostic investigations

The history of a sore throat 14 days before the onset of acute nephritis was consistent with a diagnosis of post-streptococcal GN. Serum antistreptococcal O titre (ASOT) was elevated and serum concentration of the third complement component (C3) was low, indicating complement activation, and was consistent with the presumed diagnosis. In this disease, the renal lesion represents an immunological reaction to nephritogenic antigens in the microorganism responsible for the sore throat.

The patient was referred to a nephrologist who arranged a renal biopsy (Fig. 7.2). On light microscopy, all glomeruli were infiltrated with neutrophil leucocytes and there was proliferation of mesangial and endothelial cells. Electron microscopy showed large electron-dense deposits lying between the podocytes of the visceral glomerular epithelial cells and the glomerular basement membrane. Immunofluorescence microscopy was positive for IgM, IgA and C3 in a granular capillary wall pattern. (A renal biopsy is

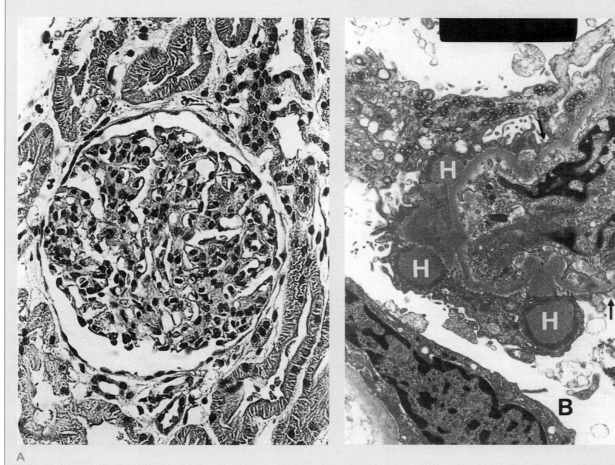

A

B

Fig. 7.2
Renal biopsy of the patient with post-streptococcal glomerulonephritis. (A) Light microscopy showing proliferation of intrinsic glomerular cells and infiltrating neutrophil leucocytes. (B) Electron microscopy showing large immune deposits ('humps' H) projecting into the Bowman's space (B) between the glomerular basement membrane (*) and glomerular epithelial cell (arrows). (C) Immunofluorescence microscopy showing coarse granular pattern for IgG along the glomerular capillary wall.

Glomerulonephritis and the acute nephritic syndrome box 3 continued

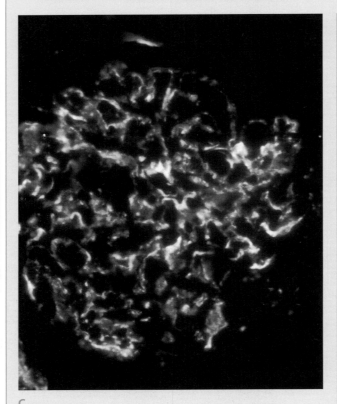

C

Fig. 7.2
Continued

frequently not necessary in this situation because the clinical and other laboratory features can be highly suggestive of the diagnosis and the long-term prognosis is usually good.)

The results of these diagnostic investigations lead to several questions which will be answered in the following sections of this chapter:

① Which serological tests are necessary to establish the diagnosis and classification of GN?

② Which renal biopsy features are useful or necessary to classify GN?

③ What insights do these features give to the pathogenesis of the renal lesion?

ledge of pathogenesis and the overlapping morphological characteristics of many types of GN.

GN may be initiated by an immune response to an exogenous antigen such as a microbial product (including streptococcal products as in the current case) or to an endogenous antigen (such as DNA with systemic lupus erythematosus; SLE). Less commonly, it may be initiated by an autoimmune response to a renal antigen, such as a component of the glomerular basement membrane in Goodpasture's syndrome (Figs. 7.4A and 7.5). The antibodies involved in these responses may form the basis for diagnostic serological tests for these diseases (see Table 7.3). A number of other effector mechanisms involving leucocytes, platelets, complement, coagulation factors and humoral products of intrinsic and infiltrating cells, act in concert with these immune mechanisms to cause glomerular injury.

When the antigen forms part of a circulating immune complex or is deposited in the kidney (e.g. on the glomerular capillary wall) to form an immune complex *in situ*, the immunofluorescence pattern is discontinuous or granular (Fig. 7.4B). In this case, corresponding electron-dense deposits are seen with electron microscopy. This pattern is seen, for example, in membranous GN, post-streptococcal GN and SLE. In most cases it is unclear whether the immune complex forms primarily in the circulation or in the kidney.

In contrast, when the antibody is directed against an intrinsic renal antigen, the immunofluorescence pattern is continuous or linear, as seen in Goodpasture's syndrome (Fig. 7.4A). In the latter situation, there should be no electron-dense deposits seen with electron microscopy.

Whether or not immune complex formation leads to the development of GN depends on numerous factors, including the nature of the antigen, the size of the complex, the antibody, the clearance of complexes by phagocytic cells, and other glomerular haemodynamic, cellular and humoral influences (Fig. 7.5).

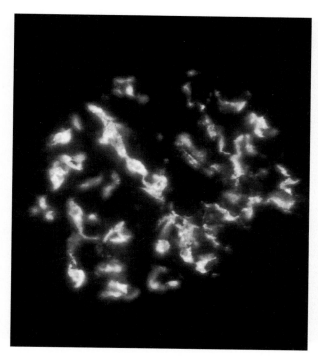

Fig. 7.3
Immunofluorescence of renal biopsy from a patient with IgA disease, showing positive immunofluorescence for IgA in a mesangial distribution. Contrast this with the 'capillary wall' distribution in Figs 7.2(C) and 7.4.

Table 7.4
Clinical and pathological differences between post-streptococcal glomerulonephritis (GN) and IgA disease

	Post-streptococcal GN	IgA disease
Antecedent pharyngitis	Yes, 10–14 days	Yes, 0–4 days
Acute nephritis	Yes	Yes
Other presentations	No	Yes*
Recurrence	No	Yes
Long-term prognosis	Excellent	Variable
Diagnostic tests		
Serological	Low C3, positive ASOT	–
Renal biopsy	Glomerular neutrophil infiltration (LM)	Mesangial IgA (IF)[†]
	Subepithelial electron-dense deposits (EM)	Mesangial electron-dense deposits (EM)

ASOT, antistreptococcal O titre; LM, light microscopy; EM, electron microscopy; IF, immunofluorescence microscopy. *Other presentations of IgA disease include macroscopic haematuria, nephrosis (uncommon), hypertension, chronic renal failure. ([†]See Fig. 7.3.)

Table 7.5
Important causes of acute nephritic syndrome

Primary
 Post-streptococcal glomerulonephritis
 Postinfective glomerulonephritis
 IgA disease*
 Mesangiocapillary (membranoproliferative) glomerulonephritis
 Crescentic glomerulonephritis
Secondary to systemic disease
 Systemic lupus erythematosus
 Microscopic polyangiitis and Wegener's granulomatosis

*Can present less commonly as a systemic vasculitis with skin, joint, gastrointestinal and renal involvement (Henöch–Schonlein purpura).

Table 7.6
Important types of glomerulonephritis (GN) and their usual clinical picture

Presentation	Primary	Secondary
Nephrotic syndrome	Minimal change disease Membranous nephropathy Focal sclerosing GN Mesangiocapillary GN	Diabetes mellitus* Amyloidosis* Systemic lupus erythematosus
Acute nephritic syndrome	Postinfectious GN Post-streptococcal GN IgA disease Mesangiocapillary GN	Systemic lupus erythematosus
Rapidly progressive GN	Crescentic GN	Microscopic polyangiitis Wegener's granulomatosis Goodpasture's syndrome

Asymptomatic haematuria/proteinuria can occur with almost all listed conditions. *These conditions are associated with a non-inflammatory glomerulopathy rather than a true glomerulonephritis.

Pathology of acute glomerulonephritis

The glomerulus may be altered in a limited number of ways in GN. Intrinsic cells (endothelial, mesangial and epithelial) may proliferate; circulating leucocytes may infiltrate; platelets may accumulate; mesangial matrix may expand; the glomerular basement membrane may change; and scarring may develop.

A hallmark of severe disease is the development of a glomerular crescent, which is a cellular, fibrinous and,

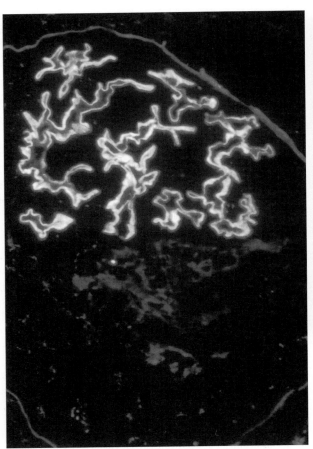

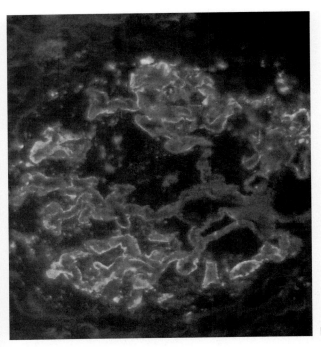

Fig. 7.4

Immunofluorescence pattern of renal biopsy specimen of glomerulonephritis initiated by: (A) autoimmune response to glomerular antigen (linear), and (B) immune response to circulating or planted extrarenal antigen (granular). Half of the glomerulus in (A) is replaced by a glomerular crescent which is not immunofluorescent. In both (A) and (B) the immunofluorescence is in a glomerular capillary wall distribution.

Glomerulonephritis and the acute nephritic syndrome box 4

Outcome

The patient received antihypertensive therapy and a loop diuretic to control fluid accumulation. Within a period of weeks his serum creatinine returned to normal, and his oedema and hypertension resolved. After 6 months his urinary sediment was inactive.

Thus, the patient's acute nephritis settled without specific treatment of the renal inflammation. But does this apply to other forms of acute nephritis?

later, fibrous lesion in Bowman's space (Fig 7.6). The greater the size and the number of crescents, the more severe the disease. Crescents may be seen in many forms of GN and, when large and numerous (in more than 50% of glomeruli), they are associated with a rapidly progressive clinical course in certain forms of vasculitis and in primary crescentic GN (see Table 7.6).

Outcome of glomerulonephritis

Given the fact that glomerulonephritides presenting with an acute nephritic picture may have a guarded prognosis, it is logical to ask about the natural history in this particular patient, and whether treatment could alter the clinical course.

See box 4

The outcome of acute GN varies greatly with the type of disease. In diseases in which the inciting antigen or event disappears spontaneously (as in the current case) or with treatment, the renal disease may resolve. In some circumstances, such as IgA disease and SLE, the disease may smoulder on or recur. When the disease remains active, smoulders on or recurs, the

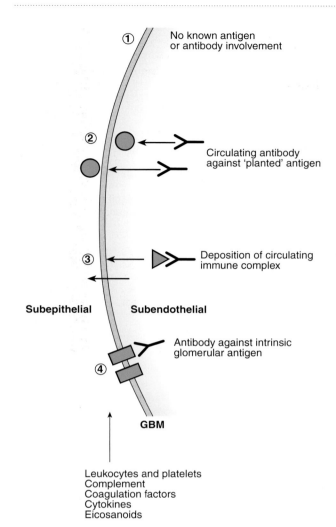

Fig. 7.5
Schematic representation of immunopathogenetic mechanisms of acute glomerulonephritis and the influence of other cellular and humoral mediators. Antigens may be deposited on the glomerular basement membrane before antibody deposition or as part of circulating antigen–antibody complexes, or may be self-antigens (usually modified) in the glomerular basement membrane.

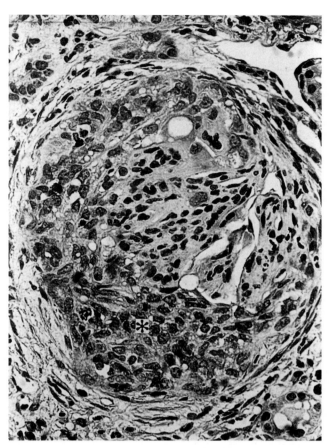

Fig. 7.6
Cellular crescent (*) occupying three-quarters of the circumference of a glomerulus and compressing the glomerular tuft.

tendency is for progressive renal scarring and renal failure to occur over a variable period of time.

Clinicopathological correlations in glomerulonephritis

No current system of classification lends itself well to the study of GN and so understanding the condition can be a daunting task. Thus, medical students should limit their study to that of the most common and/or clinically important diseases. These are listed in Table 7.6.

Some primary and secondary glomerulonephritides are usually associated with the nephrotic syndrome, as discussed in Chapter 6. Other glomerulonephritides, such as postinfectious GN and IgA disease, may present with an acute nephritic syndrome, while others, such as SLE and mesangiocapillary GN, may present with acute nephrosis or nephritis. As mentioned above, it is important to recognize the rare cases of rapidly progressive GN as they require emergency treatment.

Some important diagnostic features of the glomerular pathology in these diseases are listed in Table 7.7. These characteristic morphological and immunological features are sufficient to allow a definitive histological diagnosis to be made in the majority of cases. Further discussion of each condition included in Table 7.7 is beyond the scope of this text.

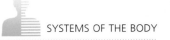

7

GLOMERULONEPHRITIS AND THE ACUTE NEPHRITIC SYNDROME

Table 7.7
Principal diagnostic glomerular appearances of important types of glomerulonephritis (GN)

	Light microscopy	Electron microscopy	Immunofluorescence
Minimal change disease	Negative	Diffuse foot process fusion	Negative
Membranous nephropathy	Thick GCW without glomerular hypercellularity	Subepithelial EDD ('lumps')	Finely granular, CW
Focal sclerosing GN	Focal segmental GS	Diffuse foot process fusion	IgM (segmental)
Mesangiocapillary GN	Thick GCW with glomerular hypercellularity	Subendothelial EDD, mesangial interposition	CW Ig and C
Postinfectious/post-streptococcal GN	Hypercellular glomerulus	Subepithelial EDD ('humps')	CW Ig and C3
IgA disease	Mesangial proliferation	Mesangial EDD	Mesangial IgA
Diabetes mellitus	GS	Thick GBM, mesangial expansion	CW pseudolinear
Amyloidosis	Variable Negative birefringence with Congo Red stain	Amyloid fibrils	–
Systemic lupus erythematosus	Various patterns	EDD – multiple sites	CW and mesangial, Ig, C3,Cl$_q$
Rapidly progressive GN	Crescents	Variable	CW negative or granular or linear

C, complement; CW, capillary wall; EDD, electron-dense deposits; GBM, glomerular basement membrane; GCW, glomerular capillary wall; GS, glomerular sclerosis.

Self-assessment case study

Joe Shapiro, an 18-year-old man, presented to his local practitioner with macroscopic haematuria. Three days before his presentation he had had a sore throat. At the ages of 15 and 16 years he had had a similar episode of macroscopic haematuria.

After studying this chapter you should be able to answer the following questions:

① Explain how urinary examination would help to narrow the differential diagnosis in this case.

② Based on the other clinical features, what is the most likely diagnosis?

③ What other clinical features are required to make a diagnosis of 'the nephritic syndrome'? What is the pathogenesis of each feature?

④ What are the main renal histopathological features of this disease?

Answers see page 148

Self-assessment questions

① What are the diagnostic clinical features of the acute nephritic syndrome? Describe their pathogenesis.

② List three conditions causing acute glomerulonephritis (GN) in which the serum concentration of complement components C3 or C3 and C4 may be reduced.

③ Which diagnostic serological tests are also involved in the immunopathogenesis of SLE, Wegener's granulomatosus, Goodpasture's syndrome, hepatitis B and C respectively?

④ Describe five clinical features which may be used to distinguish post-streptococcal GN from IgA disease.

⑤ List three ways in which antibodies may be associated with the glomerular basement membrane in acute GN.

Answers see page 149

DIABETIC NEPHROPATHY AND CHRONIC RENAL FAILURE

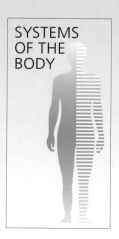

SYSTEMS
OF THE
BODY

Chapter objectives

After studying this chapter you should be able to:

① Understand the natural history of diabetic nephropathy.

② Discuss the common causes of chronic renal failure.

③ Describe the presentation and natural history of chronic renal failure.

④ Appreciate the progressive nature of chronic renal failure.

⑤ Discuss the main consequences of chronic renal failure and their pathogenesis.

⑥ Understand the principles of treatment of patients with chronic renal failure.

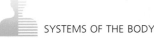
Introduction

Diabetes mellitus, both insulin- and non-insulin-dependent, is an increasingly common cause of chronic renal failure. For example, in Australia and New Zealand, which have the most reliable national statistics on **end-stage renal failure**, it now accounts for more than 25% of patients commencing dialysis or receiving a renal transplant. The incidence of diabetic nephropathy as a cause of end-stage renal failure is similar in Europe and even higher in the USA. In some ethnic groups the incidence is 40% or more.

Whatever the cause of chronic renal failure, once a certain level of renal dysfunction has been reached, renal disease tends to progress towards end-stage. We understand some, but not all, of the reasons for this progression. Renal failure has effects on almost all organ systems of the body and, as the renal dysfunction progresses, so these effects take on more clinical significance.

In this chapter we will discuss chronic renal failure and its consequences using an illustrative case of progressive renal failure due to diabetic nephropathy.

See box 1.

Presentation of chronic renal failure

The development of diabetic renal disease in this patient was not surprising, as she already manifested other evidence of diabetic microvascular complications in the form of diabetic retinopathy requiring laser photocoagulation. Microvascular complications tend to affect multiple organs concomitantly, and it would be quite unusual for a patient to develop diabetic retinopathy without coexisting nephropathy. Thus, in this patient the presentation is typical of someone with diabetes mellitus as the cause of chronic renal failure. By the time her serum creatinine was measured, she already had moderate renal failure. However, a diagnosis of chronic renal failure may be made at any time during the course of the disease. This may range from early in an asymptomatic patient following the detection of serum biochemical or urinary abnormalities to very late in a patient with few symptoms. The range of presentations of chronic renal failure is shown in Table 8.1.

Note that in this patient there were several clinical features suggesting that salt and water were being retained as a consequence of low glomerular filtration rate (GFR). Thus, hypertension, raised jugular venous pressure, pulmonary rales and oedema were manifestations of expanded extracellular fluid and plasma volumes. Another factor contributing to her oedema

---

Diabetic nephropathy and chronic renal failure box 1

Diabetes mellitus and renal impairment

Raylene Tomlein is a 35-year-old woman who has had insulin-dependent diabetes mellitus since the age of 23 years. At age 30 years diabetic retinopathy was first diagnosed and she has received regular laser photocoagulation for this since then. She first noticed mild ankle swelling at age 32 years and this slowly increased in severity. For 2 years before the current presentation she had been on antihypertensives. Her blood pressure was 155/90. There was mild peripheral oedema and her jugular venous pressure wave was visible 3 cm above the clavicle at 45°. There were bibasal pulmonary rales. Otherwise, her physical examination was normal.

Urinalysis was positive for protein (+++) and blood (trace). Urinary protein excretion was *4.5 g/24 h. Serum creatinine was elevated at *0.29 mmol/L. Ultrasound examination showed echogenic kidneys of symmetrically reduced bipolar length.

This patient had clinical features (oedema, hypertension) which suggested that her renal disease may have been present for at least 2 years. This raises the following important questions:

① How can we differentiate acute from chronic renal failure?

② How does chronic renal failure present?

③ What is the significance of her other clinical features, namely diabetic retinopathy, hypertension and proteinuria?

These issues will be discussed below.

(*Values outside normal range; see Appendix.)

Table 8.1
Presentations of chronic renal failure

Asymptomatic serum biochemical abnormality
Asymptomatic proteinuria/haematuria
Hypertension
Symptomatic primary disease
Symptomatic uraemia
Complications of chronic renal failure

---

was hypoalbuminaemia resulting from a heavy proteinuria (see Chapter 6).

The natural history of chronic renal failure tends to vary according to the aetiology. For example, the typical clinical course for a patient with insulin-dependent diabetes mellitus (IDDM) who develops chronic renal failure (as some 40% do) is illustrated in Fig. 8.1. After about 5 years of IDDM, microalbuminuria develops (albumin excretion below the range usually detected by dipstick urinalysis). Overt proteinuria then develops over the next few years followed by progressive renal impairment which leads, after another 5 years or so, to end-stage renal failure. The course tends not to be quite as predictable in patients with non-insulin dependent diabetes mellitus (NIDDM).

Differentiating acute and chronic renal failure

Renal failure is defined as a reduced GFR, which causes the kidneys to lose the ability to excrete nitrogenous wastes such as urea and creatinine; this leads to an increase in their concentration in the serum (uraemia). Certain clues help to differentiate an acute reversible increase in serum creatinine concentration (acute renal failure) from a chronic irreversible rise (chronic renal failure) (see Chapter 5 and Table 8.2). In the current patient, the long history and the reduction in renal size on ultrasonography (Fig. 8.2) indicate a chronic process. Similarly, a low haemoglobin concentration is typical of chronic rather than acute renal failure.

Stages of chronic renal failure

Chronic renal failure may be divided into different stages depending on the GFR (Table 8.3). Although arbitrary, such a division is useful in that it predicts the severity of clinical and biochemical derangements.

A patient may present at any stage of the disease. When the GFR is only mildly reduced (for example, greater than 75 mL/min) and the disease is not clearly progressive, a term such as mild renal impairment may be used. End-stage renal failure, on the other hand, may be defined by the need for dialysis therapy or renal transplantation to sustain life.

Causes of chronic renal failure

The major causes of chronic renal failure are listed in Table 8.4. Glomerulonephritis forms the largest group and, amongst the glomerulonephritides, IgA disease is the most common cause of end-stage renal failure in most western communities, accounting for 25% of cases in this category. Diabetes mellitus, as in the current patient, is the second most common cause. Analgesic nephropathy, once the second most common cause in Australia and New Zealand, is becoming increasingly uncommon. Amongst elderly patients, chronic renal failure caused by renovascular disease is being diagnosed more frequently.

Pathology of diabetic nephropathy and chronic renal disease

The renal pathological features of chronic renal disease consist of a mixture of changes typical of the primary disease and those which are common to chronic renal disease of all types. As the disease progresses, the disease-specific changes become less obvious and, in

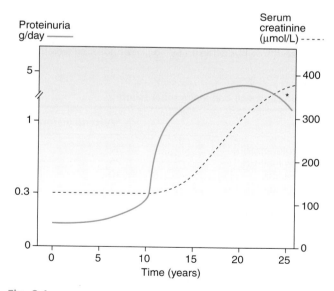

Fig. 8.1

Typical clinical course of patient with insulin-dependent diabetes mellitus who develops nephropathy.
*Proteinuria often falls late in chronic renal failure as glomerular filtration rate becomes severely impaired.

Table 8.2
Differentiation of acute and chronic renal failure

	Acute	*Chronic*
History	Short (days–weeks)	Long (months–years)
Haemoglobin concentration	Normal	Low
Renal size	Normal	Reduced
Renal osteodystrophy*	Absent	Present
Peripheral neuropathy†	Absent	Present

*Osteodystrophy is bone disease. †Peripheral neuropathy is disease or dysfunction of nerves supplying the limbs and peripheral tissues.

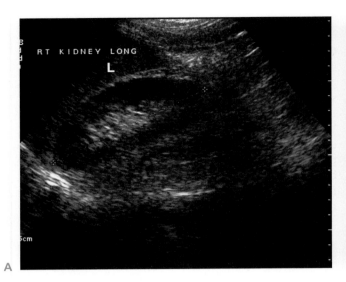
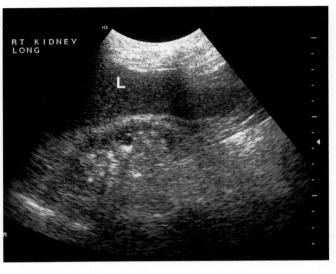

Fig. 8.2
Renal ultrasonography is useful in differentiating acute and chronic renal failure. (A) Normal-sized kidney of acute renal failure. Note that the normal kidney appears darker (less echogenic) than the adjacent liver (L). The kidney is 10.95 cm in bipolar length between markers. (B) Small, echogenic kidney of chronic renal failure. Note that a scarred kidney is brighter (more echogenic) than normal, and therefore less easy to distinguish from surrounding structures. The kidney is 7.36 cm in bipolar length.

Table 8.3
Stages of chronic renal failure

Stage of chronic renal failure	GFR* (mL/min)	Symptoms of uraemia or its complications	Serum biochemical derangements	Comment
Mild renal impairment	> 75	None	None	Not clearly progressive
Mild	50–75	None	Subtle	Early bone disease commences
Moderate	25–50	Mild	Mild	Anaemia starts
Severe	10–25	Moderate	Moderate	Salt and water retention evident
End-stage	< 5–10	Severe	Severe	Dialysis or renal transplantation necessary

*See Chapter 5 for a discussion of normal GFR (approximately 100 mL/min) and how it is affected by age, sex and body weight.

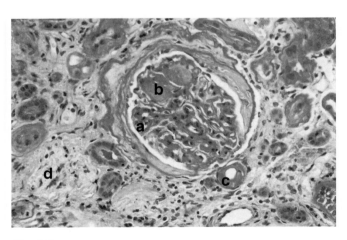

Fig. 8.3
Photomicrograph illustrating features of diabetic nephropathy. Note (a) the thickening of glomerular capillary walls, (b) nodule formation, (c) hyaline thickening of the arteriolar wall, and (d) interstitial scarring.

Table 8.4
Common causes of end-stage renal failure

	*Percentage incidence
Glomerulonephritis	30
Diabetes mellitus	25
Hypertension	10
Polycystic kidney disease	5
Vesicoureteric reflux	5
Analgesic nephropathy	5
Unknown	10
Other	10

*Approximate incidence in Australia and New Zealand (Source ANZDATA Registry): these are representative of data for other developed countries.

kidneys from patients with advanced disease, the histopathological changes become non-specific.

Early diagnostic changes in diabetic nephropathy include glomerular basement membrane thickening and expansion of the mesangium, and hyaline thickening of the afferent and efferent arterioles (Fig. 8.3). Usually there is superimposed hypertensive and sometimes infective damage (thickening of small arteries and arterioles, and interstitial inflammatory cells and scarring, respectively).

Advanced chronic renal disease is characterized by progressive scarring of glomeruli (glomerulosclerosis) and tubulointerstitium (tubular atrophy and interstitial inflammation and fibrosis).

Diabetic nephropathy and chronic renal failure box 2

Disease progression

Over the next few years Raylene's renal impairment continued to worsen slowly. She became progressively lethargic, due mainly to the development of anaemia. Her blood pressure became more difficult to control, as did her oedema. She developed mild pain in the long bones of her lower limbs, as well as generalized pruritus. On one occasion she presented with sudden shortness of breath, thought to be because of myocardial ischaemia. Her feet became numb, and a 2-cm ulcer developed on the plantar surface of her right hallux (big toe).

The progressive decline of renal function invites the following questions:

① Why does this happen?

② Can anything be done to prevent it?

The patient's symptoms were thought to be caused by complications of uraemia, affecting her bone marrow, bones, skin, central and peripheral blood vessels and peripheral nerves. In the next section, complications and consequences of chronic renal failure will be discussed.

Main consequences of chronic renal failure

The manifestations of chronic renal failure are protean, and affect every organ system of the body. They arise because the kidneys fail to perform their usual excretory, regulatory, metabolic and biosynthetic functions. The current patient developed many of these problems.

The uraemic syndrome refers to the composite clinical picture arising from concurrent appearance of many of these manifestations, but in particular those arising from the failure to excrete nitrogenous compounds (such as urea) and other 'uraemic toxins', many of which remain poorly defined. In general, there is a poor correlation between the systemic concentration of most of these substances and uraemic symptomatology. In particular, anorexia, nausea and vomiting are common uraemic symptoms, but drowsiness, lethargy, pruritus (itch), neuropathy and pericarditis can be seen when the condition is advanced.

It is sometimes difficult to differentiate symptoms of the primary disease (in this case diabetes mellitus) from those of renal failure, either because the symptoms are non-specific or because both diseases cause similar organ damage. For example, both diabetes and renal failure can be complicated by myocardial and peripheral ischaemia, and by peripheral neuropathy. Shared symptoms may thus arise earlier in the course of diabetic chronic renal failure than would be the case with other primary diseases.

Hypertension occurs mainly because of failure to excrete salt and water adequately. The resulting expansion in extracellular fluid volume triggers release of a natriuretic hormone from the central nervous system as a compensatory measure, but this also acts as a peripheral vasoconstrictor. Other contributing mechanisms may include increased renin (and therefore angiotensin) production by the scarred and ischaemic kidney, and reduced renal production of vasodepressor hormones (see Chapter 9). Peripheral oedema commonly develops and the patient may have all the features of congestive cardiac failure. While net retention of salt and water is usual, the capacity of the kidney to concentrate the urine and maximally reabsorb sodium is also impaired so, paradoxically, the patient is at risk of volume depletion in the face of restricted intake of salt and water. Overall, the range of homeostatic responses to changes in salt and water intake is greatly narrowed in chronic renal failure.

Because of efficient renal adaptive mechanisms, hyperkalaemia (arising from a failure to excrete potassium) is usually a late manifestation of renal failure. The renal adaptation consists of enhanced potassium secretion in the distal tubule. Failure to excrete acid leads to a generally mild metabolic acidosis, which contributes to renal osteodystrophy and malnutrition.

Renal osteodystrophy refers to the bone disease which occurs with chronic renal failure. It arises because of a complex interplay between calcium, phosphate, acidosis, parathyroid hormone and vitamin D (Fig. 8.4). The principal hormones involved in renal

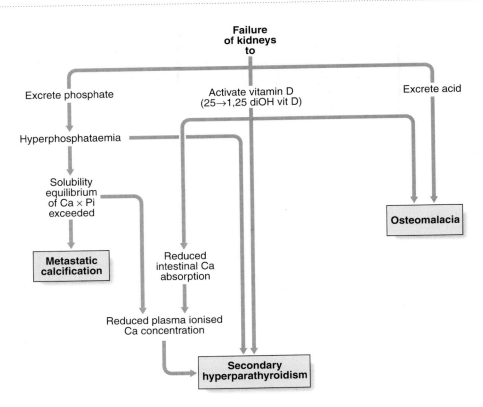

Fig. 8.4
Schema describing pathogenesis of renal osteodystrophy.

Table 8.5
Simplified physiology of parathyroid hormone and calcitriol production and action

Parathyroid hormone		Calcitriol (activated vitamin D)
		Activation
		Sterol activated by hydroxylase in kidney
		$\oplus$ by parathyroid hormone
		$\ominus$ by high plasma P_i concentration
Production		
Polypeptide with 84 amino acids secreted by parathyroid chief cells		
$\oplus$ by low plasma ionized Ca^{2+}		
$\ominus$ by high plasma ionized Ca^{2+} and calcitriol		**Action**
		$\uparrow R_{Ca}^{2+}$, $\uparrow R_{Pi}$
Action		
Kidney	$\uparrow R_{Ca}^{2+}$, $\downarrow R_{Pi}$	
	$\oplus$ 1α hydroxylase	$\uparrow$ Bone mineralization
Bone	$\uparrow$ turnover (osteoblastic formation and osteoclastic resorption)	$\ominus$ Parathyroid hormone release
Parathyroids	–	$\uparrow Ca^{2+}$ and P_i absorption
Gut	–	

R, tubular reabsorption; $\oplus$, stimulates or stimulated; $\ominus$, inhibits or inhibited; P_i, inorganic phosphate.

osteodystrophy are parathyroid hormone and activated vitamin D (calcitriol). The simplified physiology of both is summarized in Table 8.5. Reduction in serum ionized calcium concentration plays a central role. This occurs because of precipitation with elevated serum phosphate (retained because of low filtration), decreased intestinal calcium absorption because of failure of renal activation of vitamin D, and skeletal resistance to the action of parathyroid hormone. The parathyroid glands hypertrophy and secrete high levels of parathyroid hormone (secondary hyperparathyroidism) in response to the falling serum

calcium. Activation of vitamin D (cholecalciferol) normally occurs by two hydroxylation steps, the first in the liver (25-hydroxylation) to form 25-hydroxycholecalciferol, and the second in the kidney (1-hydroxylation) to form 1,25-dihydroxycholecalciferol, or calcitriol. Renal activation of vitamin D fails in chronic renal disease because of hyperphosphataemia and loss of functioning renal tissue, which prevents 1-hydroxylation of 25-OH vitamin D. The bone disease comprises a variable mix of hyperparathyroidism (causing **osteitis fibrosa cystica**), **osteomalacia** and **osteoporosis**. In addition, hyperphosphataemia leads to **metastatic calcification** in most organs, including the skin (where it can cause pruritus), blood vessels, heart and joints.

Atheromatous occlusive vascular disease can impair circulation to all organs, in particular to the heart, brain and lower limbs. Almost half the patients with end-stage renal failure die from cardiovascular events. Atheroma arises owing to multiple factors in patients with renal failure, including hypertension, smoking, dyslipidaemia and metastatic calcification.

A common early symptom in renal disease is lethargy, caused mainly by the normochromic normocytic anaemia resulting from the failure of renal erythropoietin production. Erythropoietin (or epoetin) is secreted predominantly as a glycoprotein with 165 amino acids by fibroblast-like interstitial cells in the kidney, in response to anaemia and hypoxia. Its synthesis falls as renal scarring progresses, with a consequential fall in red cell mass as its stimulatory effect on the bone marrow is lost. The reduced capacity of the blood to carry oxygen because of deficiency of erythropoietin is a major cause of morbidity in patients with renal failure, and management of this problem has been revolutionized by the availability of synthetic erythropoietin as replacement therapy. In contrast, white blood cells and platelets are normal in number, but their impaired function contributes to a predisposition to infection and a bleeding tendency, respectively.

There are many other manifestations of chronic renal failure, some common and some rare. These are summarized in Tables 8.6 and 8.7.

Progression of chronic renal failure

As illustrated by the current case, once renal impairment has become severe enough the disease tends to progress through the various stages outlined in Table 8.3 to end-stage. This occurs even when the primary

Table 8.6
Main consequences of chronic renal failure

Mechanism	Example	Consequence
Decreased excretion	Uraemic toxins, including nitrogenous wastes	Uraemic syndrome
	Salt and water	Volume overload, hypertension
	Phosphate	Hyperparathyroidism, metastatic calcification
	Acid	Metabolic acidosis
	Potassium	Hyperkalaemia
Decreased biosynthesis	Erythropoietin	Anaemia
	Activation of vitamin D	Osteomalacia, hyperparathyroidism
Altered metabolism	Dyslipidaemia	Atherogenesis
	Sex hormones	Abnormal reproductive function

Table 8.7
Organ system involvement in chronic renal failure

System	Main pathogenetic factors	Main consequences
Cardiovascular	Atheroma	Occlusive vascular disease
	Salt and water retention	Hypertension, 'congestive cardiac failure'
Bone	Secondary hyperparathyroidism	Pain, rarely fracture
	Osteomalacia	
	Osteoporosis	
Neuromuscular	'Uraemic toxins'	Sensorimotor peripheral neuropathy
		Autonomic neuropathy
		Encephalopathy
Blood	Erythropoietin deficiency	Anaemia
	'Uraemic toxins'	Impaired white cell and platelet function
Skin	Metastatic calcification	Pruritus
	Sun exposure	Skin cancer
	Anaemia and 'uraemic toxins'	Sallow complexion
Reproductive	Abnormal regulation of sex hormones	Reduced libido, impaired fertility
Gastrointestinal	'Uraemic toxins'	Anorexia, nausea, vomiting, malnutrition
Serosal	'Uraemic toxins'	Pericarditis

disease causing renal impairment has become inactive. However, if the primary disease becomes quiescent (either through natural or treatment-induced reparative processes) before renal functional impairment and scarring have become critically severe, then chronic renal failure may not be progressive.

The factors causing progression of chronic renal failure are not entirely clear, but a number of implicated factors are listed in Table 8.8. Two mechanisms receiving considerable attention over the past decade are systemic and intraglomerular hypertension, and proteinuria.

Increased glomerular hydrostatic pressure has been observed directly in several experimental models of chronic renal failure, and inferred in some forms of human chronic renal disease such as diabetic nephropathy. The resultant haemodynamic injury ('hyperfiltration') has been proposed to lead to progressive glomerular scarring.

Proteinuria is not merely a manifestation of chronic renal failure, but also an important factor leading to progressive renal scarring. It is thought that reabsorbed protein causes tubular cell damage, and also leads to tubular cell production of cytokines which incite an inflammatory and fibrogenic response in the surrounding interstitium. The net effect of these and other factors is progressive scarring of glomeruli and tubulointerstitial areas of the kidney.

This non-specific progression of chronic renal failure needs to be distinguished from separate events which may lead to superimposed acute renal failure; that is, acute-on-chronic renal failure (Table 8.9). For example, falls in extracellular fluid volume or blood pressure are commonly associated with an acute deterioration of GFR in a patient with otherwise stable chronic renal failure. When the abnormality can be corrected in a timely fashion, GFR should return to baseline. However, when the abnormality is sustained or cannot be corrected (for example, with acute renal artery occlusion in a patient with renal artery stenosis), then GFR may not improve.

Diabetic nephropathy and chronic renal failure box 3

End-stage disease

Raylene's renal failure continued to deteriorate and she was started on several different drugs to control blood pressure, fluid retention, hyperphosphataemia and acidosis. Her diet was adjusted to restrict salt, potassium, protein and fluid intake.

Three years after her presentation with chronic renal failure she was started on haemodialysis and placed on the waiting list to receive a cadaveric renal transplant.

Table 8.8
Factors causing progression of chronic renal failure

Continuing activity of primary disease
Systemic hypertension
Intraglomerular hypertension
Proteinuria
Nephrocalcinosis (dystrophic and metastatic)
Dyslipidaemia
Imbalance between renal energy demands and supply

Table 8.9
Causes of acute deterioration of renal function in patients with chronic renal failure

Recrudescence of primary disease
Complication of primary disease
Accelerated hypertension
Volume depletion
Cardiac failure
Sepsis
Nephrotoxins (radiocontrast, drugs*)
Renal artery occlusion
Urinary tract obstruction
Dietary protein load

*Including especially non-steroidal anti-inflammatory drugs and, in some situations, angiotensin-converting enzyme inhibitors and angiotensin receptor blockers (see Chapter 11).

Principles of treatment

After establishing the aetiology and severity of chronic renal failure, management is directed towards detection and treatment of factors that may cause superimposed acute renal impairment or non-specific progression, and of complications of chronic renal failure (Table 8.10). Of particular importance is the control of systemic hypertension and reduction of pro-

Table 8.10
Principles of treatment of patients with chronic renal failure

Differentiate from acute renal failure (Table 8.2)
Establish aetiology (Table 8.4)
Establish severity (Table 8.3)
Seek and treat reversible factors (Table 8.9)
Seek and treat complications (Table 8.7)
Lifestyle changes (diet, exercise, cease smoking, avoid polypharmacy)
Seek and treat factors causing progression (Table 8.8)
Planned transition to dialysis and transplantation

teinuria, for the reasons explained above. The various fluid and electrolyte and metabolic disturbances of chronic renal failure may respond well to dietary manipulation and drugs. For example, restriction of excessive dietary protein, salt, potassium, water and saturated fats may all be necessary at some stage. Hyperphosphataemia, metabolic acidosis and sodium retention may be treated with phosphate binders (such as oral calcium carbonate), sodium bicarbonate supplements, and loop diuretics, respectively. Erythropoi-etin and calcitriol may be given to replace deficiencies of those hormones. Smoking has been shown unequivocally to worsen atheromatous disease as well as progression of renal disease, and should be avoided, especially in diabetics.

In the majority of patients, chronic renal failure follows a predictable course. Thus, continuing surveillance for treatable complications and a planned transition to end-stage renal failure therapy (dialysis and transplantation) is possible and desirable.

Self-assessment case study

A 39-year-old woman with a 20-year history of insulin-dependent diabetes mellitus was found to have an elevated serum creatinine. She had had moderate nocturia for the past 4 or 5 years, and swelling and numbness of her feet for 2 years. Fundoscopy revealed changes of background and proliferative diabetic retinopathy. Her ankle jerks were absent and she was moderately tender on digital compression of her tibiae. Her blood pressure was elevated.

After studying this chapter you should be able to answer the following questions:

① What is the most likely explanation for nocturia?

② If she were to have had a renal biopsy 10 years previously, what would have been the likely histopathological features?

③ Why are her ankle jerks absent?

④ What is the explanation for her tender tibiae?

⑤ The patient also complained of weakness, and conjunctival pallor was found. What is the likely explanation?

Answers see page 149

Self-assessment questions

① Which of the following features suggests chronic rather than acute renal failure?
(a) Nocturia for several months
(b) Anaemia
(c) Small echogenic kidneys
(d) Bone pain
(e) Intact ankle jerks

② List the following clinical features in order of their appearance as glomerular filtration rate falls in progressive chronic renal failure.
(a) Oedema
(b) Anaemia
(c) Need for dialysis to sustain life
(d) Asymptomatic bone disease.

③ List the following causes of chronic renal failure according to their incidence in developed countries (most to least common):
(a) analgesic nephropathy
(b) diabetes mellitus
(c) polycystic kidney disease
(d) glomerulonephritis
(e) hypertension.

④ List the major factors which lead to secondary hyperparathyroidism in chronic renal failure.

Answers see page 149

HYPERTENSION AND THE KIDNEY

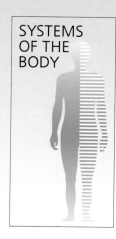

SYSTEMS
OF THE
BODY

Chapter objectives

After studying this chapter you should be able to:

① List some physiological determinants of the arterial blood pressure and explain the role of the kidney in regulating these factors.

② Discuss some mechanisms whereby abnormalities of the kidney may lead to hypertension (both essential and secondary forms).

③ Describe the pathology involved in end-organ damage due to hypertension.

④ Outline the principles of clinical and laboratory assessment of a patient presenting with hypertension.

⑤ Describe the mechanisms of action of the major classes of antihypertensive drugs.

⑥ Give the principles of management of a patient with renovascular hypertension.

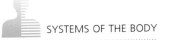
Introduction

Arterial hypertension is the most prevalent chronic disorder of western populations. If untreated, it can result in a wide spectrum of morbidity and premature mortality and, as such, its prevention and treatment are major goals for health care systems.

The kidney is involved both as a causative factor and as an organ of target damage in hypertension, and this chapter will outline some of its physiological and pathological features in relation to hypertension. The subject is a very large one and the discussion here will necessarily be selective.

See box 1.

Determinants of normal blood pressure and role of the kidney

In its simplest form, the haemodynamic description of the systemic circulation can be reduced to the statement that the mean arterial blood pressure (BP) is the product of the cardiac output (CO) and the total peripheral resistance (TPR), i.e.

$$BP = CO \times TPR$$

The cardiac output itself is the product of the stroke volume times the heart rate, where the stroke volume is determined by the left ventricular filling volume and the force of contraction. While a very wide range of physiological variables can influence blood pressure through one or other of these parameters, and the relationship between them is in fact very complex, these formulae suggest a number of levels at which the function of the kidney may impact upon the final level of the blood pressure. Some of these mechanisms are illustrated in Fig. 9.1.

The two main variables to be considered are the extracellular fluid volume (which relates directly to the cardiac output) and the degree of vasconstriction of the arterial bed (which determines the total peripheral resistance). Many aspects of renal function impinge on one or both of these variables. The following are some examples.

- Anything causing a reduction of glomerular filtration rate (GFR) will lead to retention of salt and water, with consequent volume expansion.

Hypertension and the kidney box 1

A case of deteriorating blood pressure control

Ross Schneider is a 72-year-old man who presents to his local doctor with 3 weeks of increasing headaches. He also mentions having been generally unwell for several months, with tiredness and increasing breathlessness on exertion. He is known to have had mild hypertension for over 25 years, but his blood pressure has been well controlled over this period of time, his current medication being the diuretic indapamide 2.5 mg daily. However, he has been living overseas with his son for the past 9 months and, during this period, has not had his blood pressure checked as regularly as usual. His past history also includes peripheral vascular disease, manifested 2 years previously by episodes of **claudication** in both calves on walking up hills. This symptom had eased after he stopped smoking and no further investigation or treatment had been performed.

His family history includes hypertension in his father and one of his two sisters, and ischaemic heart disease which affected his father in his fifties. Mr Schneider is a retired postal officer who smoked about 20 cigarettes per day from age 20 to 70 years. He drinks four or five beers (300-ml glasses) per day. He takes no medications other than his blood pressure tablets and says he complies strictly with these.

On examination he looks rather tired and has a pulse rate of 90 beats/min. His blood pressure is 210/100, taken in the right arm in the seated position, and this is unchanged after 5 min of rest. The apex beat is found to be displaced 2 cm lateral to the mid-clavicular line, and is thrusting (pressure-loaded) in character. Cardiac auscultation reveals a systolic ejection murmur and a loud aortic component of the second heart sound. A few soft **crepitations** are heard in the base of both lung fields. The abdomen is normal to palpation but, on auscultating over the right upper quadrant, a prolonged systolic **bruit** is heard. Peripheral pulses are difficult to feel below the popliteal in both legs. The optic fundi show thickening of arteriolar walls and **arteriovenous nipping**. Urinalysis shows protein + and no other abnormalities.

Two main issues arise for discussion from this presentation.

① What was the basis of Mr Schneider's original history of hypertension?

② What has occurred to cause his blood pressure control to be dramatically impaired at this presentation?

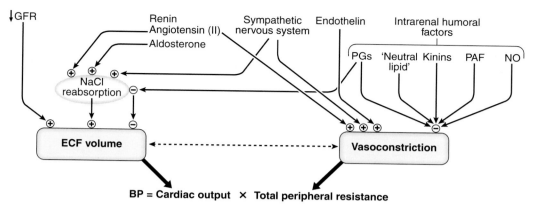

Fig. 9.1

Renal mechanisms involved in blood pressure control. Note that many interactions exist between the factors included on this schematic diagram. While extracellular fluid (ECF) volume and vasoconstriction are shown here as independent parameters, there is direct interplay between these factors, as discussed in the text. GFR, glomerular filtration rate; NO, nitric oxide; PAF, platelet-activating factor; PG, prostaglandins; + indicates a stimulating or enhancing influence, − indicates an inhibiting or suppressing effect.

- Excessive salt reabsorption by the renal tubules will also lead to increased extracellular fluid (ECF) volume.
- Activation of the renin–angiotensin–aldosterone system has the capacity to influence both variables: angiotensin II is a potent vasoconstrictor and also enhances proximal sodium reabsorption, while aldosterone stimulates distal nephron sodium reabsorption.
- The sympathetic nervous system likewise has dual actions: noradrenergic innervation of arteriolar vessels throughout the body leads to vasoconstriction and an increase in total peripheral resistance, while noradrenergic nerve endings around the proximal tubule stimulate sodium and water reabsorption at that site.
- The endothelium-derived peptide endothelin is a potent vasoconstrictor, and levels are elevated in renal failure.
- The renal prostaglandins are one of a number of locally acting signalling mechanisms influencing renal function in relation to hypertension. In this case, endproducts such as prostaglandin E_2 actually promote antihypertensive effects within the kidney, both by inhibiting salt and water reabsorption and hence promoting volume loss, and also by causing vasodilatation within the kidney and elsewhere.
- A number of other vasodilator systems have been identified within the kidney: these include a 'neutral lipid' identified in the renal medulla, the renal kinin system resulting in formation of the vasodilator bradykinin, as well as platelet-

activating factor, nitric oxide and other endothelial-based dilator systems.

It is important to emphasize that there is no simple relationship between disturbances in these factors and the generation of sustained arterial hypertension. Perturbations in any one system tend to be compensated by changes in other systems, and the critical role of central nervous system pathways modulating baroreceptor reflexes must be taken into account. Furthermore, a primary change in one major parameter, such as the ECF, can lead to secondary changes in the state of peripheral vasoconstriction, so that the final pattern of haemodynamic disturbance is different from that which triggered the initial blood pressure rise.

Pathogenesis of essential hypertension

These considerations may be relevant to the pathogenesis of so-called 'essential' hypertension, in which a specific underlying cause for increased blood pressure cannot be defined in identifiable pathology in any organ system. This pattern, which would match the initial hypertensive history of our patient Mr Schneider, is associated with a family history of hypertension and the development of an increased blood pressure in the affected subject during the third to fifth decade of life. While the precise pathogenesis of this condition has not been definitively established (and indeed a variety of physiological disturbances are capable of leading to the endpoint of sustained hypertension), one plausible scenario is shown in Fig. 9.2.

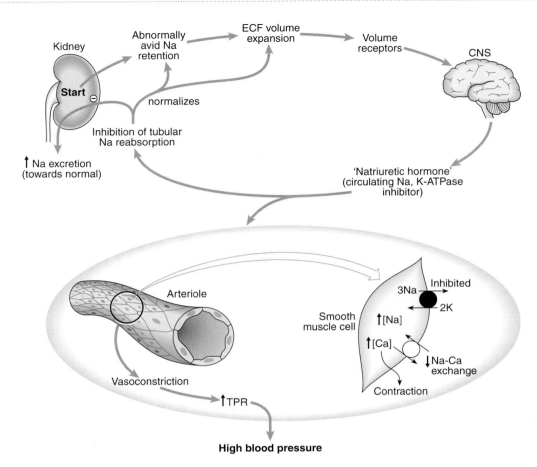

Fig. 9.2
Chronic volume expansion and hypertension: a model for essential hypertension? CNS, central nervous system; ECF, extracellular fluid; TPR, total peripheral resistance.

In this model, which is consistent with the findings of some clinical studies and a number of animal models, a primary inherited abnormality in renal salt retention is proposed, involving an overly avid sodium reabsorption mechanism in one or more segments of the nephron. This would lead to a phase of initial ECF volume expansion, which is later replaced by increased peripheral vasoconstriction and normalization of the ECF volume. One plausible mechanism whereby this haemodynamic change may occur involves the detection of the early volume expansion by volume receptors whose afferent signals into the central nervous system result in the release of a natriuretic hormone. Such a substance has been defined in the circulation during volume expansion, with properties like those of the natural **glycoside** ouabain, namely that it acts as an inhibitor of membrane-bound Na,K-ATPase. Inhibition of this enzyme in the renal tubules results in impaired sodium reabsorption and hence increased urinary excretion of salt and water, serving to correct the expanded ECF volume towards normal. However, inhibition of the same enzyme in

smooth muscle cells within arteriolar walls results in an increase in intracellular sodium concentration which, by slowing the activity of a sodium–calcium exchanger in the muscle cell membrane, leads to an increase in intracellular calcium. This change triggers activation of the contractile mechanism of the smooth muscle fibres, leading to generalized vasoconstriction and an increase in total peripheral resistance, corresponding with the observed pattern of steady state haemodynamics in established hypertension.

While speculative, the schema described above does accord with much of the available data about renal and circulatory changes observed during the generation and maintenance of hypertension. It also gives a framework for considering other factors known to predispose towards hypertension, whether or not there is another pathologically definable cause. A list of such risk factors is provided in Table 9.1.

Among the non-modifiable risk factors is a positive family history of hypertension. While this can not universally be associated at this stage with a specific genetic defect, a number of rare inherited syndromes

Table 9.1
Risk factors for development of high blood pressure (other than specific secondary forms of hypertension)

Non-modifiable
  Family history
    Inherited predisposition to essential hypertension
    Specific inherited conditions (e.g. Liddle's syndrome, metabolic syndrome)
Potentially reversible
  Lifestyle factors
    Obesity (± sleep apnoea)
    Excessive salt intake
    Excessive alcohol intake
    Physical inactivity
  Iatrogenic
    Oral contraceptive pill use
    Use of non-steroidal anti-inflammatory drugs
    Steroid therapy
    Excessive use of topical or systemic vasoconstrictor medications

Hypertension target organs

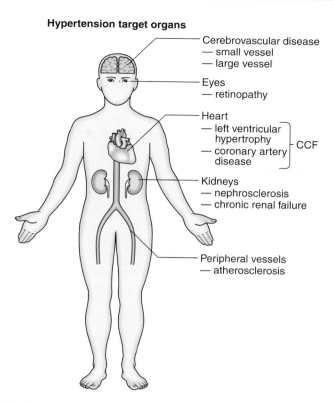

Fig. 9.3
End-organ damage in hypertension. CCF, congestive cardiac failure.

have been defined which do fit in with the above model for essential hypertension involving primary renal volume retention. Of recent interest is the definition of the cause of hypertension in Liddle's syndrome, in which blood pressure elevation early in life is associated with evidence for volume expansion (suppressed renin and aldosterone levels). Here overexpression of the epithelial sodium channel in the apical membrane of the cortical collecting duct epithelium has been identified and linked to a specific gene defect. Similar but more subtle causes of increased tubular sodium avidity may underlie a wider spectrum of patients with familial hypertension. For example, in the 'metabolic syndrome', in which hypertension is associated with obesity and insulin resistance, an increase in proximal tubular sodium–hydrogen exchange has been found.

Of the non-genetic factors, at least some of the reversible factors may operate through enhanced renal sodium retention. Certainly the epidemiological and clinical evidence relating to a correlation between salt intake and hypertension is suggestive of a primary role for volume expansion (at least in genetically predisposed individuals). The hypertension of common obesity may also be caused by volume expansion, possibly mediated by high insulin levels which act to enhance proximal sodium reabsorption. Renal salt retention is also implicated in the hypertension associated with a variety of medications, including oestrogens, non-steroidal anti-inflammatory drugs which interfere with prostaglandin synthesis, and corticosteroids.

ECF volume expansion also has an important role in the genesis of a number of forms of secondary hypertension; these are discussed later in this chapter.

The pathology of hypertension

Whatever the cause of a sustained increase in arterial blood pressure, a number of forms of end-organ damage result from this haemodynamic change. As shown in Fig. 9.3, the kidneys are included among these target organs.

The fundamental pathology associated with hypertension is based on structural changes in the terminal radicals of the arterial tree, namely the small muscular arteries and arterioles. The repetitive mechanical stress associated with hypertension causes changes in all layers of the vessel wall, particularly in the media layer, where smooth muscle hypertrophy results in a thickening of the arterial wall with concentric narrowing of the lumen. The internal elastic lamina becomes reduplicated and interrupted, and hyaline degeneration may occur in focal areas of the media where a glassy eosinophilic material accumulates. These changes, found in so-called 'benign' hypertension, are replaced in the more accelerated and severe variant known as 'malignant' hypertension by a more destructive severe form of vascular wall pathology, the characteristic lesion being that of fibrinoid necrosis. In all forms of sustained hypertension, the intima layer is also damaged and undergoes a proliferative response, which in larger vessels is associated with acceleration of the process of **atherosclerosis**.

These vascular lesions lead to various grades of ischaemia in the principal target organs, namely the brain, the heart and the kidney. Small vessel changes in the brain are reflected in the optic fundi, where progressive stages of vascular damage and retinal ischaemia can be observed directly (hypertensive retinopathy). In the heart, myocardial ischaemia develops, and is aggravated by the development of left ventricular hypertrophy as a result of the chronic pressure load on that chamber. Within the kidney, ischaemia is manifested initially by wrinkling of the glomerular basement membrane. Hypertrophic and hyaline changes develop in the afferent arterioles, resulting in progressive atrophy and ultimately sclerosis of glomeruli (Fig. 9.4). In severe and neglected hypertension this can lead to end-stage renal failure, a not uncommon outcome despite current antihypertensive treatment (see Chapter 8). Ischaemic changes also affect the tubules, which undergo atrophy, associated with interstitial inflammatory changes progressing ultimately to fibrosis. Eventually the kidney as a whole undergoes contraction with a finely scarred surface ('nephrosclerosis').

It is clear that the kidney has an especially complex relationship to arterial hypertension. As mentioned previously (and to be developed further below), it is directly implicated in the aetiology and pathophysiology of some forms of hypertension, notably those in which definable renal disease provides the primary

trigger for the development of high blood pressure. Equally, however, it is an important end-organ of damage from hypertensive vascular disease, thereby setting up a vicious cycle of further aggravation of the hypertension (Fig. 9.5). Intervention in this cycle by vigorous therapy to lower the blood pressure and protect the kidney is thus a crucial task for those caring for these patients.

See box 2.

Principles in the management of hypertension

In a patient presenting for the first time with hypertension, management consists of three general steps:

1. Confirmation of the persistence of hypertension on multiple observations following modification of reversible lifestyle factors (see Table 9.1).
2. Baseline investigations to assess end-organ damage (particularly in the heart and kidney), to quantitate other vascular risk factors (particularly plasma lipid profile), and to screen for major causes of secondary hypertension as clinically appropriate (see below).
3. Initiation of pharmacological treatment.

This staged approach can be accelerated in situations in which the blood pressure is severely elevated at presentation (>160/100) or where there is clinical evidence of organ-threatening complications such as heart failure, renal impairment or neurological symptoms or signs. In practice, in the absence of specific clinical clues, the 'screening' investigations in the second step can be limited to urinalysis to detect renal parenchymal disease and plasma biochemistry to detect renal failure or electrolyte changes suggestive of endocrine hypertension. Further investigations are initiated

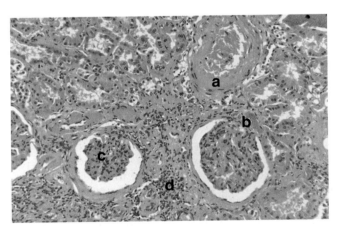

Fig. 9.4
Microscopic pathology of the kidney in 'benign' essential hypertension. Note (a) the hypertrophied arterial walls and (b) hyaline degeneration of the afferent arteriole . One glomerulus (c) has undergone ischaemic contraction and there is interstitial fibrosis and inflammation (d).

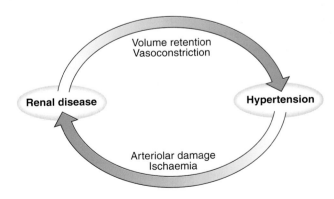

Fig. 9.5
The kidney in hypertension: villain (cause) or victim (effect)?

Hypertension and the kidney box 2

Initial investigations

Mr Schneider's physical examination (see box 1) revealed clear evidence for end-organ damage consistent with hypertensive effects. The displaced and prominent left ventricular impulse suggests the presence of left ventricular hypertrophy with some cardiac enlargement, and the pulmonary crepitations and recent history of breathlessness are consistent with early left ventricular failure. The history of claudication and finding of poor distal pulses in the legs suggest the development of peripheral vascular disease, while the finding of Grade II hypertensive retinopathy (thickened retinal arteriolar walls with arteriovenous nipping) implies hypertensive effects on small arterioles. The detection of + proteinuria on urinalysis is consistent with hypertensive damage to glomeruli.

The initial investigations performed on Mr Schneider reveal the following results.

Plasma biochemistry:
Sodium 135 mmol/L
Potassium 4.1 mmol/L
Chloride 99 mmol/L
Bicarbonate 29 mmol/L
*Urea 9.2 mmol/L
*Creatinine 0.18 mmol/L.

These levels had been normal when last checked 3 years previously.

Random blood glucose is 6.8 mmol/L and the lipid profile is normal. A chest X-ray shows a moderately enlarged heart (principally the left ventricle) and bilateral pulmonary congestion. Electrocardiography shows evidence of left ventricular hypertrophy with non-specific ST segment changes.

These data were interpreted as evidence for renal and cardiac damage resulting from his hypertension.

While waiting for these initial investigation results, Mr Schneider's doctor initiated some changes in his therapy, having made the assessment that he had experienced a marked deterioration in his level of blood pressure control. He urged the patient to discontinue all alcohol intake, to reduce his salt intake, to continue with his diuretic medication and to commence taking prazosin 2 mg three times daily. He asked to review him in 3 days time. He explained that he suspected that some new problem had arisen causing his hypertension to become exacerbated, and that he thought some further investigations would be required.

Issues for further consideration at this point include:

① What clues are there as to the cause of Mr Schneider's deterioration in blood pressure control?

② What are the appropriate next steps in his management?

(*Values outside the normal range; see Appendix.)

---

when abnormalities are detected on these preliminary tests, taken in conjunction with clinical information.

The selection of an appropriate antihypertensive medication depends on properties of the available agents (including cost), patient characteristics and co-morbid conditions, guided by information from relevant published clinical trials. A brief summary of some key features of the available drugs is given in Table 9.2. Frequently, drugs are given in combination to reduce side effects and oppose secondary compensations which can reduce the effectiveness of a single agent.

Deterioration in blood pressure control

When a patient who has been stabilized on an antihypertensive treatment regimen experiences a deterioration in blood pressure control, as did Mr Schneider, a number of possibilities must be considered (Table 9.3). The patient's adherence to the recommended treatment regimen must always be checked since poor compliance is a relatively frequent phenomenon, especially when the medications used are associated with unwelcome side effects. Occasionally, the inadvertent coprescription of an interacting medication may be the cause; the best example here is commencement of a non-steroidal anti-inflammatory drug which promotes salt and water retention and will elevate the blood pressure in predisposed individuals. Occasionally, there has been a progressive slide into poor lifestyle habits which raise the blood pressure, such as weight gain beyond ideal body weight or excess intake of salt or alcohol.

An important consideration in an older patient, however, is the possibility that a form of secondary hypertension has become superimposed on what was originally essential hypertension.

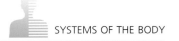
Table 9.2
Overview of main classes of antihypertensive drugs

Class	Prototype drug(s)	Advantages	Disadvantages
Diuretics	Chlorothiazide	Useful in coexistent CCF, adjunctive action with other agents	Electrolyte/metabolic side effects, allergies
Beta-blockers	Atenolol (beta-1 selective)	Beneficial in IHD	Fatigue, insomnia; may worsen asthma, heart block, PVD, lipids
Alpha-blockers	Prazosin	Metabolically neutral	Postural hypotension
Calcium channel blockers*	(a) Verapamil (b) Nifedipine	All useful in angina (best used in slow-release preparations)	(a) May cause constipation, worsen heart block/CCF; (b) Cause flushing, oedema
ACE inhibitors	Captopril	Beneficial in CCF, reduce proteinuria, conserve K	Cough, angio-oedema, reduce GFR in renal artery stenosis
AII receptor blockers	Losartan	As for ACE inhibitors, but less cough	
Centrally acting drugs	Methyldopa, clonidine		Drowsiness, depression
Direct acting vasodilators	Hydralazine, minoxidil		Reflex tachycardia, oedema

ACE, angiotensin-converting enzyme; A II, angiotensin II; CCF, congestive cardiac failure; GFR, glomerular filtration rate; IHD, ischaemic heart disease; PVD, peripheral vascular disease. *Representative drugs are shown for the two main classes of calcium channel blockers: (a) the non-dihydropyridines, and (b) the dihydropyridines.

Table 9.3
Causes of deterioration in blood pressure control

Poor treatment adherence (compliance)
Commencement of interacting medications (e.g. NSAIDs)
Lifestyle changes (weight gain, excessive salt or alcohol intake)
Superadded secondary hypertension (especially renovascular or renal parenchymal disease)

NSAIDs, non-steroidal anti-inflammatory drugs.

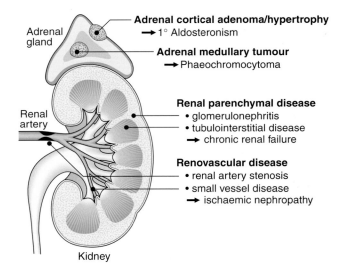

Fig. 9.6
Principal causes of secondary hypertension.

Adrenal gland

Adrenal cortical adenoma/hypertrophy
→ 1° Aldosteronism

Adrenal medullary tumour
→ Phaeochromocytoma

Renal artery

Renal parenchymal disease
• glomerulonephritis
• tubulointerstitial disease
→ chronic renal failure

Renovascular disease
• renal artery stenosis
• small vessel disease
→ ischaemic nephropathy

Kidney

Secondary hypertension

The principal causes of secondary hypertension are illustrated in Fig. 9.6. One of these causes may be defined soon after presentation in a patient with newly diagnosed hypertension, or following a period of resistance to therapy or deterioration in blood pressure control in a patient with established hypertension. It should be emphasized that less than 10% of all hypertensive patients have hypertension secondary to a defined pathology in a specific organ system, although a higher percentage of underlying causes can be reported from clinics seeing a patient group referred for further investigation of 'difficult hypertension'. While causes other than those shown in Fig. 9.6 need to be considered in special patient groups (e.g. coarctation of the aorta in hypertensive children and pre-eclampsia in pregnant women), the most commonly encountered causes of secondary hypertension arise from conditions in the adrenal gland or the kidney.

Adrenal causes

Adrenal lesions causing hypertension may arise either in the adrenal cortex or medulla.

The adrenal cortex can be the site of an aldosterone secreting adenoma, resulting in primary aldosteronism, or Conn's syndrome. In this condition autonomous production of aldosterone by the tumour leads to sustained salt and water retention by the kidney, with volume expansion and secondary vasoconstriction which sustains the hypertensive state, as previously discussed. Frequently, this condition is accompanied by hypokalaemia, reflecting the action of aldosterone in enhancing renal potassium excretion. While a low serum potassium, usually accompanied by an elevated bicarbonate concentration, may act as a useful clue to the presence of an aldosterone excess state, these electrolyte abnormalities are not universally found in cases of primary aldosterone overproduction, and some authorities recommend screening for this condition in all patients whose hypertension is resistant to usual treatment. One screening approach depends on the measurement of plasma aldosterone and renin concentrations, using a high aldosterone : renin ratio as a signal for further adrenal investigation. Primary aldosteronism can also arise from hyperplasia of both adrenal cortices, sometimes because of an inherited defect in adrenal corticosteroid biosynthesis.

When the adrenal adenoma or cortical hypertrophy is associated with autonomous secretion of the glucocorticoid hormone cortisol, Cushing's syndrome results, hypertension being one of the principal clinical manifestations. Other clues here are bodily **habitus** changes associated with glucocorticoid excess, accompanied by hyperglycaemia as well as hypokalaemia and alkalosis.

The adrenal medulla may also give rise to tumours causing hypertension, in this case phaeochromocytoma, secreting the catecholamines adrenaline (epinephrine), noradrenaline (norepinephrine) and related metabolites. These tumours can also arise in neural crest-derived tissue outside the adrenal gland. Characteristically they are associated with labile hypertension, with spasms of vasoconstriction and organ ischaemia related to bursts of catecholamine release. However, a significant proportion of these tumours are accompanied by sustained hypertension without such dramatic episodic changes in the peripheral circulation. Investigation is based on an index of suspicion, leading to 24-h urine collections for measurement of catecholamines and their metabolites, followed by CT imaging of the adrenal gland. Radioisotope scans with specialized tracers (e.g. MIBG; *meta*-iodobenzguanine) can be useful in localizing extra-adrenal phaeochromocytomas. The pathophysiology of the hypertension in this condition relates to intense catecholamine-induced vasoconstriction rather than primary volume expansion. The cornerstone of treatment before operative removal of the tumour is effective alpha-blockade using agents such as phenoxybenzamine.

Renal causes

The kidney can be the cause of secondary hypertension by one of two fundamental mechanisms: via activation of the renin–angiotensin system in renal ischaemia due to renovascular disease, or through non-renin-dependent mechanisms in renal parenchymal disease, both in its early stages and in end-stage renal failure.

The mechanisms involved in the various forms of renal hypertension are best illuminated through some classic experiments first performed by Goldblatt over 60 years ago (Fig. 9.7).

When the renal artery supplying one kidney of an animal is clipped so that the lumen is reduced by more than 70%, the animal develops hypertension. The mechanism of the initial phase of blood pressure rise is dependent on the activation of secretion of renin from the clipped kidney, largely because of the fall in perfusion pressure in the afferent arterioles beyond the obstructed artery (see Chapter 2). Within the first few weeks after production of this lesion, the blood pressure can be normalized by agents interfering with the action of angiotensin II, verifying that vasoconstriction produced by this peptide is the main mechanism for the hypertension. The ECF volume does not undergo significant change in this phase, partly because the reduction in sodium excretion from the clipped kidney is compensated by an increase in sodium excretion from the unclipped kidney. This is because of the effect of the increased blood pressure in the unclipped kidney to inhibit salt and water reabsorption in proximal tubules on that side (so-called 'pressure natriuresis'). After some months, however, the increased blood pressure becomes resistant to the action of angiotensin inhibition, but does respond to a reduction of ECF volume. This is because of the long-term effects of sustained hypertension on the blood vessels of the unclipped kidney, where obliterative changes lead to glomerular damage and reduced excretion of salt and water from that side. That is, the initial vasoconstriction-mediated hypertension has been replaced by a volume-dependent pattern.

When a similar experiment is performed in an animal in which one of the kidneys has been removed, clipping the renal artery of the remaining kidney also leads to development of hypertension, but in this case both the early phase and the longer term phase of hypertension are dependent on an expanded ECF volume. This is because, despite the ischaemia which would otherwise trigger renin release, the overall reduction in total GFR means that volume retention occurs early in the model, counteracting the stimulus for renin release and triggering hypertension through secondary vasoconstriction via mechanisms described earlier in this chapter. This model provides a basis for understanding the hypertension of advanced renal insufficiency ('renoprival' hypertension), in which volume expansion is nearly always present.

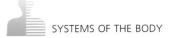

9

HYPERTENSION AND THE KIDNEY

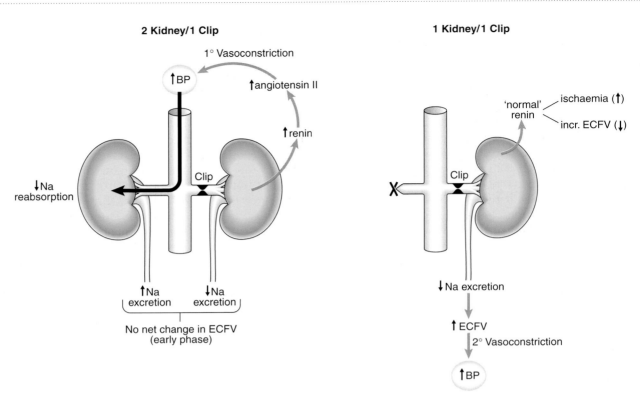

Fig. 9.7
Pathophysiology of renovascular hypertension (Goldblatt models). The two experimental models shown here represent extreme illustrations of the role of vasoconstriction (early phase of two kidney/one clip model) and volume expansion (one kidney/one clip) in the generation of hypertension during renal ischaemia (see text for details). BP, blood pressure; ECFV, extracellular fluid volume.

Renal artery stenosis

Renal artery stenosis occurs in man in one of two main pathological forms.

Fibromuscular dysplasia is a congenital condition in which the development of the media or adventitia layer of the renal artery (and sometimes other arteries) is abnormal, leading to an irregular narrowing of the lumen, often in a 'beaded' pattern. Typically affecting young women in the second or third decade of life, this is one of the classic causes of secondary hypertension in a young patient and, when unilateral, is usually detected in the phase of high renin release from the affected kidney, corresponding to the initial phase of two kidney/one clip Goldblatt hypertension. Surgical intervention to correct the stenosis frequently results in restoration of normal blood pressure and protection of renal function.

The more common cause of renal artery stenosis is that due to atherosclerosis, affecting patients in older age groups. In this condition the atherosclerotic pathology, which may also affect other vascular beds, involves one or both renal arteries, frequently producing a relatively focal stenosis (Fig. 9.8). While there is often no special clue to the presence of this underlying lesion, the clinician's index of suspicion that stenosis is present is raised by the following:

- The relatively sudden appearance of hypertension in an older person.
- The development of resistance to usual antihypertensive medications or an abrupt deterioration in blood pressure control in a patient with previously stable hypertension (as in our current case).
- Severe hypertension in an older patient associated with progressive deterioration of renal function.

Careful clinical, biochemical and radiological analysis is necessary to define the presence of renal artery stenosis in selected patients, and the pathophysiological assessment and appropriate management of such patients is frequently a complex matter. Three

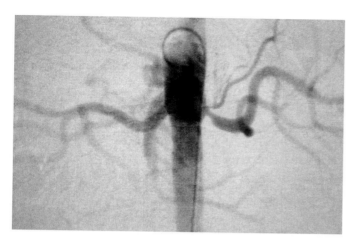

Fig. 9.8
Intra-arterial digital subtraction arteriogram showing atheromatous renal artery stenosis on the left side in a 60-year-old woman with severe hypertension.

Table 9.4
Methods of renal artery imaging

Technique	Comments
Digital subtraction angiography	Intra-arterial method provides gold standard; intravenous approach lacks adequate resolution
	Requires use of contrast agent (may reduce GFR)
Spiral CT angiography	Good 3D images; uses intravenous contrast (often high volumes required)
Magnetic resonance angiography	Avoids contrast agent; accurate only for main (proximal) vessels, expensive, limited availability
Renal artery Doppler–ultrasound scan	Operator-dependent; variable sensitivity/specificity
Radionuclide renography with captopril	Poor anatomical resolution but sensitive detection of functional stenosis via GFR effects

GFR, glomerular filtration rate.

basic components are involved in the overall assessment:

- What is the morphology of the lesions in the renal artery (or arteries)?
- What is the role of the renal artery stenosis in the pathogenesis of the patient's hypertension at this time?

- What is the influence of the renal arterial disease on overall renal function?

A number of imaging modalities, summarized in Table 9.4, may be used to define the anatomy of the renal arteries. While intra-arterial digital subtraction arteriography (Fig. 9.8) is the gold standard for definition of renal artery lesions, recent technical advances have made alternative less invasive procedures such as magnetic resonance angiography attractive alternatives.

One procedure which gives poor anatomical definition but potentially useful functional information is the captopril renogram. The uptake of a tracer isotope by both kidneys is compared before and after administration of a single dose of the angiotensin-converting enzyme (ACE) inhibitor captopril. The rationale for this test depends on the fact that, in the ischaemic kidney, the GFR in individual nephrons is maintained by the vasoconstrictor action of locally produced angiotensin II on the efferent arteriole. Thus, reduction of angiotensin II synthesis by captopril leads to an abrupt fall in tracer filtration in the kidney affected by significant renal artery stenosis. The sensitivity of this test is reduced in the presence of renal impairment.

The functional effect of the stenosis can be indirectly assessed by comparing the renin concentration in blood samples taken directly from the renal vein draining each kidney: an increase in renal vein renin on the affected side of greater than 1.5 times the contralateral kidney is suggestive of significant ischaemia. While this investigation has some capacity to predict the renin dependence of hypertension in the early phase of renovascular hypertension, its utility is limited, both by technical factors and because hypertensive vascular disease has frequently supervened in the unstenosed kidney by the time many such patients are investigated (equivalent to the late phase of two kidney/one clip Goldblatt hypertension). Indeed, intervention to improve the blood flow into kidneys affected by atherosclerotic renal artery stenosis is sometimes justified by the need to preserve long-term renal function, regardless of the mechanism by which the renal artery disease has contributed to the patient's hypertension.

Renal parenchymal disease
Hypertension in renal parenchymal disease has multiple possible origins. In the phase before advanced loss of renal function has occurred, one important factor may be the loss of vasodilator substances generated normally by healthy renal tissue (including the

'neutral lipid' from the renal medulla). This may lead to unopposed systemic vasoconstriction. However, as renal functional impairment progresses, the dominant mechanism is undoubtedly retention of salt and water as a result of the inadequate GFR, leading to expansion of the ECF volume and hypertension through secondary vasoconstrictive mechanisms (discussed previously). Thus, the great majority of patients approaching end-stage renal failure, or on dialysis, have volume-dependent hypertension which can be difficult to control until salt and water is removed from the ECF by diuretics or a form of dialysis.

In a minority of patients with advanced renal disease (< 10%), the pathological processes within the kidney cause it to act as an ongoing source of renin release, producing hypertension via angiotensin-induced vasoconstriction. In individual patients, activation of the sympathetic nervous system appears to play a role in the pathogenesis of hypertension in renal failure, and in these cases high circulating levels of catecholamines are found.

See box 3.

While the precise pathophysiology involved in the hypertension associated with renovascular disease is rarely defined clearly in an individual patient, the pattern illustrated by Mr Schneider's case is fairly characteristic of the situation in atherosclerotic renal artery stenosis. While ischaemia and renin release may be involved relatively early in the pathological process, the contralateral kidney is soon affected by hypertensive arteriolar disease, superimposed on any pre-existing vascular or parenchymal changes (this is a major cause of the fall in GFR in this clinical setting). Thus, while correction of the renal artery stenosis cannot be expected to cure the hypertension altogether, it can result in improved ability to control the blood pressure (reduced medication requirements), and may help to preserve renal function both in the kidney affected by the stenosis and also in the contralateral kidney through better blood pressure control. While the risks associated with open surgical procedures to improve renal artery flow (bypass grafting or endarterectomy) can make the decision to intervene difficult, more recent closed procedures involving balloon angioplasty with stent placement have made intervention more viable for a larger number of patients.

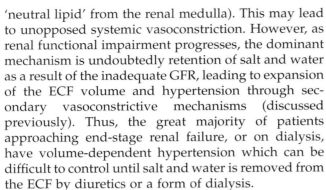

Hypertension and the kidney box 3

Further investigations and management

Three factors in Mr Schneider's case led his doctor to initiate further investigation for renal artery stenosis. First, a bruit over the upper abdomen had been heard on clinical examination, suggestive (but not diagnostic) of critical narrowing in a renal artery or other branch of the abdominal aorta. Second, he had recently developed clinical evidence for significant peripheral vascular disease, suggestive of a widespread process of advanced atherosclerosis. Third, his serum creatinine had risen over recent years, suggesting some cause of impaired glomerular perfusion.

After referral to a consultant nephrologist, a number of further studies were performed which confirmed this suspicion. A renal ultrasound demonstrated that the right kidney was 3 cm smaller in longitudinal axis than the left kidney, and a renal artery Doppler ultrasound study indicated wave forms consistent with stenosis near the origin of the right renal artery. A radionuclide scan indicated reduced uptake and excretion of tracer on the right side, with a further drop in right-sided perfusion after a 25-mg dose of captopril.

With these preliminary data in hand, Mr Schneider went on to undergo an intra-arterial digital subtraction angiogram of his renal arteries. A 90% stenosis in the proximal segment of the right renal artery was demonstrated, with only minor luminal irregularities in the left renal artery, but significant atheromatous disease in the abdominal aorta. At the same procedure, the right renal artery lesion was dilated by balloon angioplasty and a short metallic **stent** was implanted to maintain luminal patency at the end of the procedure. Mr Schneider tolerated the procedure well. The day after this intervention his plasma creatinine rose to *0.23 mmol/L, but over the next few weeks it fell to a value of *0.15 mmol/L, where it remained for several months of follow-up. His blood pressure became rather easier to control, although it still required the coadministration of indapamide plus prazosin 1 mg b.d.

(*Values outside the normal range; see Appendix.)

Self-assessment case study

A 52-year-old woman is referred for assessment of resistant hypertension. She has had raised blood pressure for only 5 years, during which time a variety of medications have been tried to control the blood pressure, with limited success. Treatment with a thiazide diuretic was partly effective, but produced severe hypokalaemia (plasma potassium *2.4 mmol/L), and had to be discontinued. Even in the absence of diuretic treatment, the plasma potassium is generally in the range 2.9–3.6 mmol/L. Currently, imperfect blood pressure control has been achieved using the beta-blocker atenolol, 50 mg daily, plus the ACE inhibitor enalapril, 10 mg twice daily.

After studying this chapter you should be able to answer the following questions:

① What possible cause of secondary hypertension is suggested by this story?

② What further investigation would you recommend?

③ What form of imaging may be helpful in defining an underlying adrenal neoplasm?

④ If primary aldosteronism is confirmed, what are the treatment options?

Answers see page 149

Self-assessment questions

① By what mechanisms does the renin–angiotensin–aldosterone system act as an effector arm in the control of systemic blood pressure?

② Name some lifestyle factors which have been proven to be risk factors for the development of hypertension.

③ Name three organs which are major targets for tissue damage during uncontrolled hypertension.

④ Why does hypertension develop when blood flow into one kidney is restricted by renal artery disease?

⑤ Name five categories of antihypertensive drugs, citing a potential disadvantage or complication of therapy in each case.

Answers see page 150

URINARY TRACT OBSTRUCTION AND STONES

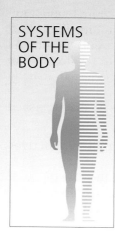

SYSTEMS
OF THE
BODY

Chapter objectives

After studying this chapter you should be able to:

① Recognize the principal causes of loin pain.

② Recognize the principal causes of haematuria.

③ Understand the pathophysiology of urinary tract obstruction.

④ Discuss the complications of urinary tract obstruction.

⑤ Discuss the investigation and principles of treatment of urinary tract obstruction.

⑥ Describe some common types of urinary tract stones and outline their forms of presentation and management.

Introduction

Loin pain may arise because of pathology in the nerves radiating from the spinal cord, vertebral column, paraspinal and lumbar muscles, and retroperitoneal organs such as kidneys, abdominal aorta and pancreas. The simultaneous presence of haematuria strongly suggests that the loin pain is caused by pathology in the kidneys or ureters. If loin pain and/or haematuria are present, then it is necessary to consider whether urinary tract obstruction is also present. The following case history describes a patient with a renal calculus (stone) causing loin pain, haematuria and urinary obstruction.

Urinary tract obstruction and stones box 1

Loin pain and haematuria

Kevin Whiteside is a 63-year-old man who presented to the Casualty department of his local hospital with a 6-h history of right-sided pain and smoky (reddish–grey) urine. The loin pain was situated at the level of the first three lumbar vertebrae and radiated around the right side of his abdomen. After several hours it radiated further into his right testis and the upper medial aspect of his right thigh. The pain was constant and very severe. His right kidney was ballottable and very tender. (Ballottement refers to the rebound felt by the hand placed over the middle–upper quadrant of the abdomen when the fingers of the other hand tap upwards in the loin to displace the kidney.) He was afebrile, sweating and pale. His blood pressure and the remainder of his physical examination were normal. Urinalysis was strongly positive for blood.

The main features in this patient's history were the presence of severe loin pain and macroscopic haematuria. The haematuria suggested strongly that the pain originated in the urinary tract rather than other potential sites.

Differential diagnosis of loin pain and haematuria

Any back or retroperitoneal structure may give rise to back pain (Table 10.1). Pain arising from spasm of a tubular or hollow organ, such as the ureter, is referred to as colic. The severity and radiation of this patient's pain were typical of renal colic, although pain of a similar distribution could occur because of compression or involvement of a nerve root. The extension of the pain into his right groin and inner right thigh is

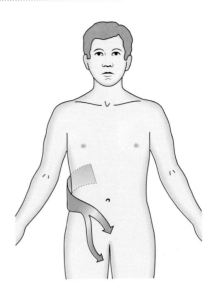

Fig. 10.1
Site of renal colic. Renal colic typically radiates from the loin around to the lower quadrant of the abdomen and the upper medial thigh on the same side.

Table 10.1
Principal sites of pathology leading to loin pain

Spinal nerve roots
Vertebral column
Paraspinal and lumbar muscles
Kidneys
Renal pelvis/ureters
Abdominal aorta
Pancreas

explained by movement of the pathology down the ureter (Fig. 10.1). Renal pain arises because of rapid stretching or inflammation of the renal capsule, whereas pain arising from the renal pelvis or ureter is caused by distension and excessive peristaltic contractions.

Macroscopic haematuria may arise from lesions anywhere within the urinary system, including the kidney itself, the renal pelvis, ureter, bladder and urethra. As few as 5×10^6 red cells per millilitre (1 microlitre of blood per millilitre of urine) can be detected visually as red-coloured urine.

Macroscopic haematuria needs to be distinguished from the following:

- Red discolouration of urine caused by certain dyes and occasional drugs.
- The presence of haem pigment in the case of intravascular haemolysis (haemoglobin from red blood cell lysis) or rhabdomyolysis (myoglobin from muscle breakdown).

- Bleeding outside the urinary tract (e.g. perineum or vagina).

The relationship of the blood to urine helps to distinguish bleeding involving the bladder or above (uniform discoloration of urine) from that arising from the urethra (blood separate or mixed with urine).

Haematuria arising from the renal parenchyma (glomeruli or interstitium) tends to be accompanied by proteinuria and casts, whereas bleeding arising from renal tumours or from lesions in the renal pelvis or below may be isolated or (particularly with infection) associated with pyuria (white blood cells in the urine). Moreover, most red blood cells arising from renal parenchymal lesions have an abnormal morphology (best appreciated by phase contrast microscopy), whereas those from renal tumours or more distal lesions have a normal biconcave appearance (Table 10.2). Red cells may also be damaged by urine of high osmolality (which causes cell shrinkage) or low osmolality (causes cell swelling and haemolysis). With brisk bleeding there may be frank blood with little urine.

Macroscopic haematuria arising from tumours tends to be painless, whereas that arising from calculi or infection is usually associated with pain. Occasionally, crystals (microcalculi) can cause pain and macroscopic haematuria. Renal calculi and urological tumours are discussed in more detail later in this chapter.

See box 2.

Imaging of the urinary tract

As outlined in Chapter 1 (in the context of urinary tract infection), there are multiple investigations from which to choose to image the urinary tract. These are summarized in Table 10.3. Each has particular attributes so the choice depends on the suspected diagnosis and the question to be answered.

In the investigation of loin pain and macroscopic haematuria, adequate information can usually be obtained from simple investigations. As 90% of renal calculi are radio-opaque, the plain abdominal X-ray is a useful first test (see Fig. 10.2). Ultrasonography is cheap and non-invasive, and provides useful information about renal size, renal mass lesions (in particular cysts), and renal pelvic and ureteric dilatation (see Fig. 10.3).

Pathophysiology of urinary tract obstruction

The presence of renal pelvic dilatation (hydronephrosis) on the current patient's ultrasound scan indicates a partial or complete obstruction to urinary flow; there was no hydroureter, consistent with the obstruction being caused by the calculus at the level of the pelvi-ureteric junction. Stones of 1 cm or greater diameter are unlikely to pass beyond this level spontaneously. As with any hollow organ, obstruction could be due to an extrinsic, intramural or luminal lesion. Common causes of urinary tract obstruction are listed in Fig. 10.4.

The patient's age and gender and clinical setting often allow accurate prediction of the cause of obstruction. Obstruction may be bilateral, in particular with lesions of the bladder or urethra.

As a result of urinary flow obstruction, resting intra-luminal pressure rises (from 1 up to 80 mmHg) and leads to proximal functional and structural changes.

Table 10.2
Differential diagnosis of red urine

	With loin pain	Uniform discoloration of urine	Haem pigment on dipstick	Red blood cells in urine	Casts and protein in urine	Predominantly dysmorphic red blood cells
Foods and dyes (e.g. beetroot)	−	+	−	−	−	−
Drugs	−	+	−	−	−	−
Pigmenturia (haemolysis or rhabdomyolysis)	−	+	+	−	−	−
Non-urological bleeding	−	−	+	+	−	−
Urethral bleeding	−	−	+	+	−	−
Renal, ureteric or bladder tumours	−*	+	+	+	−	−
Calculi or infection	+	+	+	+	−	−
Renal parenchymal lesion (glomerulonephritis or interstitial nephritis)	±	+	+	+	+	+

*Ureteric and bladder tumours may cause pain because of obstruction.

Urinary tract obstruction and stones box 2

Obstruction

As the pain was typical of renal colic, Kevin was suspected of having a renal calculus. A plain abdominal X-ray was arranged; this demonstrated a large radio-opaque lesion lying to the right of the L2/L3 vertebrae (Fig. 10.2). An abdominal ultrasound demonstrated dilatation of the right renal pelvis (hydronephrosis) above a hyperechogenic, shadowing lesion (renal calculus) with normal thickness and echogenicity of the right kidney (Fig. 10.3).

The imaging of the patient's renal tract demonstrated a renal calculus causing blockage of urinary flow. These findings give rise to the following questions:

① What are the different modalities for imaging the urinary tract? Which are the best for a patient with a suspected renal calculus?

② Why do renal calculi occur?

③ What are the consequences of urinary tract obstruction caused by a renal calculus?

Each of these questions will be answered below.

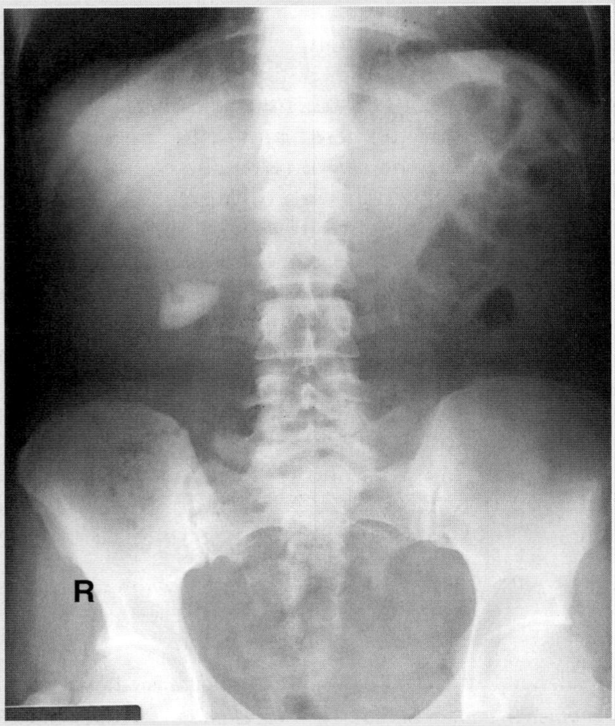

Fig. 10.2
Plain abdominal X-ray of the current patient showing a radio-opaque calculus near the second and third lumbar vertebrae on the right.

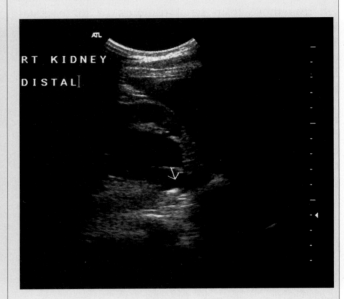

Fig. 10.3
Ultrasound scan of the right kidney of the current patient showing dilatation of the renal pelvis and an echogenic lesion (arrowed) at the pelviureteric junction, associated with an acoustic shadow beneath it. The denser an object is in relation to water the brighter it appears on ultrasound (echogenic). Note how the contents of the renal pelvis (urine) appear black, that is, non-echogenic.

Ureteral peristalsis increases in frequency and amplitude initially. The ureter and renal pelvis dilate (Fig. 10.5) and, with persistent obstruction, peristalsis diminishes and becomes disorganized, and intraluminal pressure falls.

The pressure effects are transmitted to the kidney and lead to a range of structural and functional changes (Table 10.4). As might be predicted, distal tubular function becomes compromised with impairment of the following:

- water and sodium reabsorption
- urinary concentration
- acid and potassium secretion.

After an initial phase of compensatory vasodilatation, glomerular filtration rate (GFR) and renal blood

Table 10.3
Imaging of the urinary tract

Test	Particularly useful for:	Cost
Plain abdominal X-ray	Radio-opaque calculi	+
Plain renal tomogram	Renal size and outline	+
Intravenous pyelogram*	Renal size, outline and function (nephrogram)	++
	Renal pelvis, ureter and bladder (excretory phase)	
Retrograde pyelogram*	Bladder visualization by cystoscopy**, ureter and renal pelvis	++++
Antegrade pyelogram*	Obstructed renal pelvis and ureter	+++
Ultrasonography	Renal cysts, size and pelvis	++
Dynamic isotope scan†	Renal blood flow, differential function, and outflow	++
Static isotope scan†	Renal size and scars	++
CT	Renal mass lesions, non-radio-opaque calculi	++++
Spiral CT	Renal artery anatomy	
Magnetic resonance imaging	Renal mass lesions	++++
Magnetic resonance angiography	Renal arterial flow	

*A pyelogram is an X-ray image of the renal pelvis. **Cystoscopy is an examination of the bladder performed prior to contrast injection up the ureters. †'Dynamic' isotopes (e.g. **DTPA**) are filtered and excreted by the kidney, whereas 'static' isotopes (e.g. **DMSA**) are taken up by renal cells.

A Obstruction can be intraluminal, intramural, extrinsic

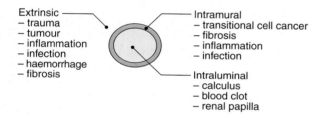

Extrinsic
– trauma
– tumour
– inflammation
– infection
– haemorrhage
– fibrosis

Intramural
– transitional cell cancer
– fibrosis
– inflammation
– infection

Intraluminal
– calculus
– blood clot
– renal papilla

B Common causes of obstruction

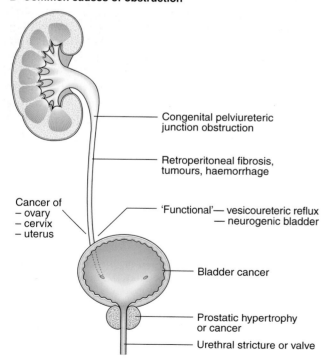

Congenital pelviureteric junction obstruction

Retroperitoneal fibrosis, tumours, haemorrhage

Cancer of
– ovary
– cervix
– uterus

'Functional'— vesicoureteric reflux
— neurogenic bladder

Bladder cancer

Prostatic hypertrophy or cancer

Urethral stricture or valve

Fig. 10.4
Sites and causes of urinary obstruction.

Table 10.4
Functional consequences of urinary tract obstruction

Reduced glomerular filtration rate
Reduced renal blood flow (after an initial rise)
Impaired renal concentrating ability
Impaired distal tubular function
   Nephrogenic diabetes insipidus
   Renal salt wasting
   Renal tubular acidosis
   Impaired potassium secretion
Postobstructive diuresis

flow fall because of a combination of the back-pressure effects and release of locally active vasoconstrictor hormones (in particular thromboxane A_2 and angiotensin II), which alter intrarenal haemodynamics (Fig. 10.6).

These functional changes may be reversible with relief of acute obstruction, or partially reversible or irreversible with prolonged obstruction, leading to renal scarring. Characteristically, with the relief of obstruction and therefore the passage of urine, the distal functional defects may become manifest clinically. This is called postobstructive diuresis, caused by an osmotic and physiological diuresis due to excretion of retained water, sodium and urea. A persistent defect in collecting duct function involving impaired aquaporin 2-mediated water reabsorption (a form of nephrogenic diabetes insipidus; see Chapter 3) contributes to postobstructive diuresis. Renal scarring occurs over a period of weeks because of the effects of pressure and the release of chemoattractant and fibrogenic cytokines, such as osteopontin and monocyte chemoattractant protein 1, and transforming growth factor β, respectively.

With unilateral, slowly progressive and/or partial obstruction, the symptoms and clinical and laboratory signs of obstruction may not be obvious.

Renal calculi

Renal calculi (stones) are a common cause of loin pain, haematuria and urinary tract obstruction. Some 90% of calculi are radio-opaque and so may be detected by plain radiography, as with the current patient.

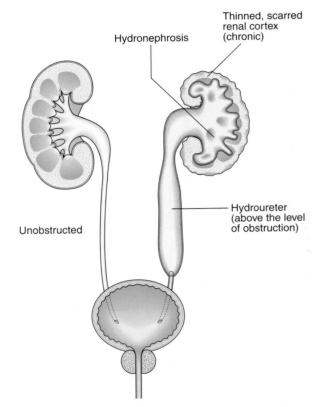

Fig. 10.5
Structural consequences of urinary tract obstruction.

Common types of renal calculi are listed in Table 10.5. An illustration of the physical characteristics of specific types of stone is given in Fig. 10.7. Urinary stasis, caused by poor urine output or obstruction, is an important pathogenic factor in the formation of most stones. Other factors relevant in particular cases include altered urinary pH, low concentration of naturally occurring stone inhibitors (e.g. citrate), infection (especially with microorganisms that split urea to form ammonia), and excess urinary excretion of the substances which form stones owing to excess dietary intake, systemic overproduction or release, and/or reduced renal reabsorption.

The current patient's calculus was causing obstruction of urinary flow, and was too large to pass to the bladder spontaneously. This raises the question of what would happen if the obstruction were not relieved, and how should the stone be treated. These issues will be addressed in the last section of this chapter.

See box 3.

Principles of treatment

With urinary tract obstruction, the main principle of treatment is to relieve the obstruction to prevent functional and structural damage to the kidney (Table 10.6). If left untreated for a period of weeks, this damage becomes irreversible. However, with superadded urinary infection the patient may become septicaemic and develop pyonephrosis (an infected obstructed kidney) with rapid renal destruction: these conditions require emergency treatment. Stones less than 1 cm in diameter may pass spontaneously, whereas larger stones require surgical intervention. Depending on their size, position and composition they may be treated with a combination of lithotripsy (to fracture the stone into fragments), endoluminal extraction (from within the urinary tract lumen) or open surgical removal.

Table 10.5
Renal calculi

Composition	Percentage	Radio-opaque	Appearance	Crystal shape	Pathogenesis
Calcium oxalate	60	+++	Small, smooth or spiky	'Back of envelope' or dumb-bell	Hyperparathyroidism, hypercalciuria, hypocitraturia, hyperoxaluria, hyperuricosuria
Calcium phosphate	20	+++	Slightly larger, more friable	Elongated	Distal renal tubular acidosis
Uric acid	< 10	–	May be large	Rhomboidal	Low urinary pH, hyperuricosuria
Struvite ($MgNH_4PO_4$)	< 10	++	Staghorn	'Coffin lid'	Infection with urease-producing microorganisms
Cystine	< 5	+	Pale yellow, may be large	Hexagonal	Cystinuria

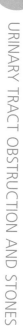

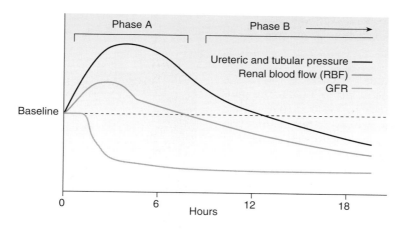

Pathophysiology of changes in —

	Intraluminal pressure	RBF	GFR
Phase A	↑ ...due to: Obstruction ↑Peristalsis	↑ ...due to: Vasodilatation —prostacyclin —prostaglandin E_2	↓ ...due to: ↑ Intratubular pressure
Phase B	↓ ...due to: Disorganised peristalsis Dilatation of tubules and ureter	↓ ...due to: Vasoconstriction —angiotensin II —thromboxane A_2	↓ ...due to: —continuing obstruction —vasoconstriction

Fig. 10.6
Functional consequences of acute urinary tract obstruction.

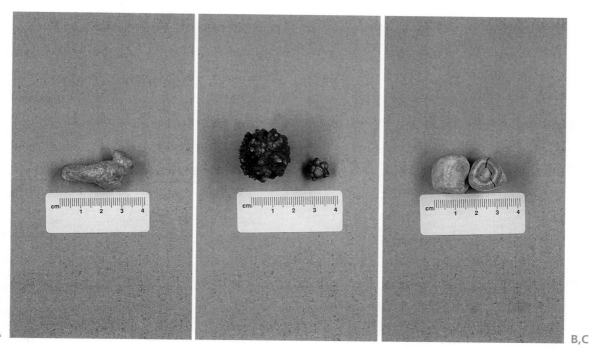

Fig. 10.7
Macroscopic appearance of renal calculi. (A) Staghorn calculus (forming a cast of the calyces and renal pelvis); (B) spiculated (spiked) stones of calcium oxalate ('mulberry' stones or 'jackstones'); (C) lamellated (layered) bladder stones, mainly of uric acid. Specimens courtesy of the Department of Urology, Concord Hospital.

Urinary tract obstruction and stones box 3

Infection and treatment

Over the next 24h the patient became febrile (39°C), with **rigors** and an increase in left loin pain. The peripheral white cell count rose to *15.0 × 10⁹/L with a predominant neutrophilia. It was felt that infection had developed proximal to the obstructing stone.

The patient was started on intravenous antibiotics and, on the same day, was taken to the operating theatre. Here the stone was manipulated by ureteric instrumentation back into the renal pelvis and a ureteric stent placed to relieve the obstruction. (A stent is a narrow tube which is placed within the ureter to maintain its patency.) Between 50 and 100mL of purulent fluid passed through the ureter when the stent was placed. The patient improved over the next few days.

Four weeks later he underwent extracorporeal lithotripsy (shattering of a calculus using external shock waves) and subsequently passed a number of stone fragments (Fig. 10.8). These were analysed and shown to consist predominantly of calcium and oxalate.

With stasis of urinary flow, microorganisms are not flushed out and can multiply. The addition of infection to the patient's clinical picture turned this into a condition which required emergency treatment.

(*Values outside the normal range; see Appendix.)

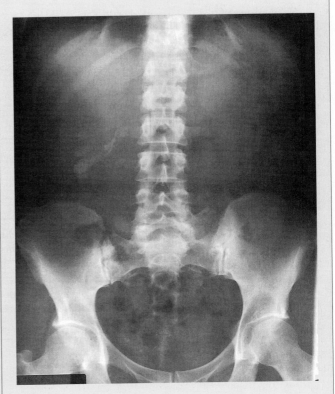

Fig. 10.8
Plain abdominal X-ray showing stone fragments after extracorporeal lithotripsy of the stone shown in Fig. 10.2.

Table 10.6
Principles of treatment of renal calculi

Emergency	Narcotic analgesics for pain relief
	Correction of fluid and electrolyte disturbances
	Intravenous antibiotics for systemic or intrarenal infection
	Relief of obstruction to treat infection and preserve renal function
Remove calculus	
Determine pathogenesis	Stone analysis
	Fluid intake and dietary history
	Family history for genetic factors
	Serum and urinary 'metabolic screen'
Prevent further calculi	Increased fluid intake (e.g. 2.5–3 L/day)
	Modification of diet
	Specific treatment of metabolic abnormality

Table 10.7
Principal malignant urological tumours in adults

	Cell type	Presentation	Differential diagnosis
Grawitz*	Renal tubular cell	Painless haematuria	Simple cysts, benign tumours
Renal pelvis, ureter, bladder	Transitional cell	Haematuria or obstruction	Other intraluminal lesions (e.g. stone, papilla, clot)
Prostate	Glandular epithelium of prostate	Haematuria, obstruction, metastatic disease	Benign prostatic hypertrophy, prostatitis

* Grawitz is a commonly used eponym for renal cell carcinoma.

Where possible, the pathogenesis of stone formation in a particular patient should be determined to guide appropriate treatment measures to prevent further stone formation. Pathogenesis can usually be inferred from a dietary history, history of fluid intake, information about familial occurrence, urinary culture, and a 'metabolic screen' of plasma and urine. The main components of the metabolic screen are determined by the usual or expected composition of the stone (see Table 10.5), and include plasma calcium and uric acid, urinary pH, calcium, uric acid, oxalate, citrate and, in some cases, cystine.

Urological tumours

Macroscopic haematuria in this patient was due to renal calculus disease, but the differential diagnosis included urological tumours. As discussed above, urinary tract obstruction may be caused by extrinsic compression from non-urological tumours, such as cervical, uterine or ovarian cancer, or from tumours of the lower urinary tract (renal pelvis, ureter, bladder and prostate). A summary of the principal types of malignant urological tumours in adults is given in Table 10.7.

Self-assessment case study

A 75-year-old man presented with inability to pass urine for 12 h. He had a 3-year history of increasing problems in passing urine (micturition). He noted difficulty in initiating micturition, a weak urinary stream and post-micturition dribbling. In the past he had had an episode of macroscopic haematuria associated with dysuria and fever. On examination of his abdomen, there was fullness and tenderness in the suprapubic area. His serum creatinine was twice the upper limit of normal.

After studying this chapter you should be able to answer the following questions:

① What is the most likely explanation for his acute history of difficulty in passing urine?

② What is the likely explanation for the previous episode of dysuria, macroscopic haematuria and fever?

③ Explain why his serum creatinine was elevated.

④ What is the best test to confirm the diagnosis?

⑤ What are the main principles of treatment in this situation, and why?

Answers see page 150

Self-assessment questions

① Abnormalities of what structures can give rise to loin pain?

② How can the red urine occurring with haemolysis be distinguished from that occurring with haematuria?

③ Describe the pathophysiology behind changes in renal blood flow and GFR during the first 24 h after acute obstruction.

④ List the chemical composition of five types of renal calculi.

Answers see page 151

DRUGS AND THE KIDNEY

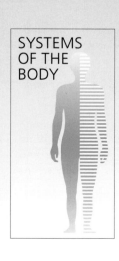

SYSTEMS
OF THE
BODY

Chapter objectives

After studying this chapter you should be able to:

① Describe the mechanisms of renal excretion of drugs in patients with normal and impaired renal function.

② Recognize characteristics of a drug that will increase its action and/or toxicity in patients with impaired renal function.

③ Identify patients in whom drug dosage should be modified in light of renal disease, changes in total body water or protein-binding which will affect the distribution or toxicity of the drug.

④ Describe the common mechanisms that underlie nephrotoxic insults to the kidneys.

⑤ Understand the natural history of the common forms of drug-induced nephrotoxicity.

⑥ Describe some preventative therapies and monitoring procedures that should be put in place before prescribing potentially nephrotoxic drugs.

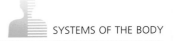

11

DRUGS AND THE KIDNEY

Introduction

Many drugs are excreted by the kidney through glomerular filtration, tubular secretion or a combination of these processes. Conjugated metabolites produced by the liver are also excreted by the kidney. Reduced renal clearances in patients with kidney disease may result in accumulation of drugs and their metabolites, with increased risk of toxicity. Renal dysfunction may also affect the distribution of the drug in the body by altering total body water, or the metabolism or protein-binding of the drug, which in turn may modify its therapeutic and adverse effects.

In addition to the effect of pre-existing renal dysfunction on drug excretion and metabolism, many drugs may themselves directly influence renal function through:

• Effects on volume status or renal haemodynamics that may alter the glomerular filtration rate (GFR).

• Accumulation of the drug or its metabolites causing direct toxicity to the kidney.

Mechanisms to 'protect' the kidney from nephrotoxic insults and to maintain cellular integrity exist, but these are likely to be impaired in the presence of chronic renal failure, which further predisposes to drug nephrotoxicity.

This chapter will discuss the factors and mechanisms influencing drug excretion by the kidneys in patients with both normal and abnormal renal function in Part A. In Part B, the physiological and cellular basis for drug-induced nephropathies will be considered.

PART A

Effect of renal impairment on drug excretion

Drugs and the kidney box 1

Too much digoxin?

Mrs Beverley Johnson is a 71-year-old woman who has been under treatment from her general practitioner for heart failure for several years. She has underlying ischaemic heart disease and suffered an acute myocardial infarction affecting the anterior wall of the left ventricle at the age of 68. Since that time, she has been treated with an angiotensin-converting enzyme (ACE) inhibitor (lisinopril 5 mg daily) and a diuretic (furosemide [frusemide] 40 mg twice daily).

Recently Mrs Johnson's condition deteriorated, with increased shortness of breath and fatigue. After admission to the local hospital's Emergency department, she was found to have developed **atrial fibrillation** and was started on digoxin 0.25 mg daily. Ten days after returning home from this admission, she called her GP to visit her because she had been experiencing increasing nausea with three episodes of vomiting since her discharge.

On examination, Mrs Johnson looks pale and uncomfortable, but is haemodynamically stable (blood pressure 130/80, pulse 86 beats/min, still in atrial fibrillation). She appears a little dry, and weighs 56 kg (usual weight 57–58 kg). The doctor checks his records, which reveal that Mrs Johnson's biochemistry (at the time of her recent admission) showed normal electrolytes, but slightly increased plasma concentrations of urea (*9.5 mmol/L) and creatinine (*0.14 mmol/L),

reflecting some renal impairment presumed to be caused by vascular disease and poor cardiac output.

The doctor now suspects that digoxin toxicity has developed, and takes blood for a serum digoxin level as well as electrolytes and renal function. He advises her to stop taking the digoxin until he gets the results.

This case raises the following questions:

① How is the kidney involved in the metabolism and excretion of drugs?

② What characteristics of a drug are likely to predict whether the kidney has a primary role in determining its plasma concentration?

③ What patient characteristics influence the metabolism and excretion of a drug under normal circumstances?

④ How and when should drug dosing be modified in the presence of renal impairment?

Before we consider the specifics of Mrs Johnson's clinical problem, it is useful to consider the general principles involved in the normal metabolism and excretion of a drug that will influence its prescription.

(*Values outside the normal range; see Appendix.)

Principles of drug dosing

The dosage of a drug and the frequency with which it is given requires an understanding of both its pharmacodynamics and pharmacokinetics. Pharmacodynamics refers to the relationship between drug dose, plasma concentration and the effect of the drug. Pharmacokinetics describes the parameters of absorption, distribution and excretion of the drug: these factors determine the dose that should be administered and the dosage interval required to maximize effectiveness of the drug and minimize side effects. Many patient-related factors will influence the pharmacodynamics and pharmacokinetics, and this should be reflected in both the dosage and timing of drug administration.

An important pharmacodynamic concept is that the response to a drug is related to its concentration, either in plasma or in tissue. The classic relationship between dose and effect is demonstrated in Fig. 11.1A. It is clear from this relationship that a minimal concentration of drug is necessary to achieve a desired effect and that once a certain level of drug is reached no further therapeutic effect is gained. However, if higher concentrations of drug are obtained then toxicity may ensue. The overlap between toxic and beneficial effects is referred to as the therapeutic index. For some drugs there is a large difference between the drug levels at which maximum efficacy is achieved and toxicity develops (Fig. 11.1B). In these circumstances, dosage modification is not generally needed in renal failure, even if the drug accumulates to high levels (e.g. penicillin). However, other drugs have a narrow therapeutic index, which means that toxicity occurs at a level close to the maximal efficacy (Fig. 11.1C). It is in these circumstances that blood levels of the drug, generally taken just before the next planned dose, are most useful to ensure that efficacy is maintained and the risk of toxicity minimized. This is the case, for example, with digoxin.

Altered pharmacokinetics in renal disease

As described above, pharmacokinetic factors determine the plasma concentration achieved after a drug is administered. These factors include the absorption of the drug, its distribution in body fluids and tissue, and its excretion. All of these steps may be altered during renal disease, although the greatest effect is on excretion.

Gastrointestinal absorption

The amount of drug absorbed from the gastrointestinal tract largely depends on the characteristics of the

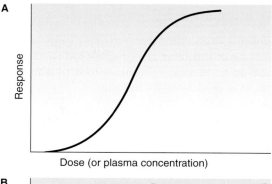

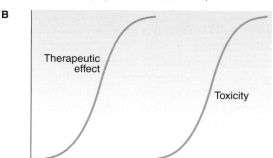

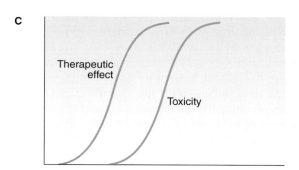

Fig. 11.1

Theoretical dose–response curves for a drug (response on *y* axis as percentage of maximum effect, dose on *x* axis as log drug concentration). (A) Basic dose–response relationship; (B) dose–response relationship for the therapeutic effect and the toxic effect of a particular drug (no overlap, i.e. wide therapeutic index); (C) dose–response relationship for the therapeutic and toxic effects of another drug (with overlap, i.e. narrow therapeutic index).

drug rather than patient-related factors. However, in patients with renal impairment, the absorption of drugs from the gastrointestinal tract may be reduced because of gastric stasis, reduced gastric acidity and concurrent treatment with phosphate-binding drugs which will also bind numerous medications (e.g. aspirin, ciprofloxacin).

Drug distribution

The volume of distribution (V_d) of a drug is defined as the volume of fluid that the drug would need to be distributed in to produce the measured plasma concentration. It is calculated as follows:

$$V_d = \frac{\text{dose of drug administered}}{\text{plasma concentration}}$$

The volume of distribution for a drug exclusively confined to the plasma approximates the plasma volume. This is likely to be the case for drugs which are very highly protein-bound. If a drug is very water-soluble, then the volume of distribution approximates body water (approximately 60% of body weight in men and 55% in women). The volume of distribution may be altered in renal failure because of fluid retention and expansion of the circulating volume. For water-soluble drugs with low protein-binding, this may reduce the effective drug concentration.

Renal failure results in accumulation of organic acids that compete with drugs for binding onto albumin and other plasma proteins. As serum albumin may be low in renal failure, an increased proportion of free drug may be available. However, the changes in protein binding rarely require a change in the loading dose of drugs, nor in the interpretation of steady state plasma drug levels, with the exception of phenytoin. In this instance the therapeutic range for total plasma concentration needs to be adjusted downward to take into account increased free drug availability.

Renal excretion

The excretion of a drug (and its clearance) is related to the volume of distribution of the drug and its half-life ($t_{1/2}$), which is the time for its plasma concentration to halve after absorption and distribution of the drug are complete. The $t_{1/2}$ of a drug may help in determining dosage interval and predicting drug accumulation. It is often important to know how long it will take before a drug reaches its full effect, i.e. its steady state concentration. The time required for any drug to achieve this steady state is four to five times its $t_{1/2}$ (Fig. 11.2A).

If the half-life of a drug is prolonged in renal failure because of a reduction in clearance, then a widening of the dosage interval is required, and the time to reach steady state may be prolonged (Fig. 11.2B). This has implications for drugs such as digoxin, which normally has a $t_{1/2}$ of 36 h, and thus steady state is reached after 1 week. However, in renal failure the $t_{1/2}$ is prolonged, and steady state may not be reached for several weeks. A corollary of this is that, where the

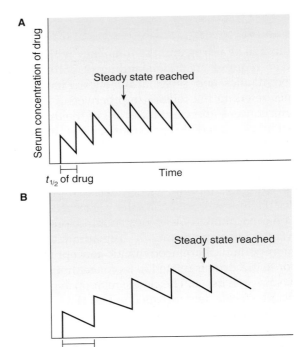

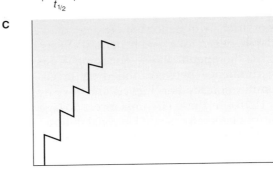

Fig. 11.2
Time course of plasma drug concentrations after repeated oral administration of the same dose at constant time intervals. (A) Drug administered at interval corresponding to its half-life of elimination ($t_{1/2}$); steady state reached in approximately five half-lives. (B) Same drug with prolonged half-life caused by reduced drug excretion in renal failure; when dose is given every (new) half-life, the time to steady state is greatly prolonged; (C) same drug given in renal failure at interval corresponding to half-life in normal renal function, resulting in rapid accumulation of drug to excessively high levels.

dosing interval is not altered, administration of the usual dose of the drug will rapidly lead to accumulation of high serum concentrations (Fig. 11.2C). This may have serious clinical consequences for drugs such as digoxin, which have a narrow therapeutic index, and both the effective dose and toxicity correlate closely with the steady state plasma concentration.

The renal excretion of a drug is determined by filtration and the net effect of tubular secretion and reabsorption.

The filtration of a drug into the urine depends largely on its molecular weight and the degree to which it is protein-bound. In general, filtration is increased with a lower molecular weight and a lesser degree of protein binding. Once filtered, lipid-soluble drugs may be passively reabsorbed from the tubular fluid down a concentration gradient to the plasma. Water-soluble drugs may be 'trapped' in the tubular fluid and excreted if no specific reabsorptive mechanism exists.

Some drugs undergo active secretion into the urine by facilitated (carrier-mediated) transport mechanisms that normally transport organic acids or bases across the proximal tubular wall. The basic cellular mechanisms involved in this secretory process are illustrated in Fig. 11.3. It has been established that, for organic acids (including many anionic drugs), the initial step in secretion is the uptake of the anion into the cell across the basolateral membrane by cotransport with sodium, which enters the cell down its electrochemical gradient (generated by the action of the basolateral Na,K-ATPase). The anion then reaches a relatively high intracellular concentration and leaves the cell down its concentration gradient into the lumen, exchanging via a countertransport carrier with another anion such as chloride. The secretory mechanism for organic bases and cationic drugs is less well defined, but probably involves a primary secretory step across the apical cell membrane, with secondary increase in uptake across the basolateral membrane. A representative list of drugs undergoing secretion by one or other of these pathways is given in Table 11.1.

Drugs undergoing transport across the tubular epithelium may be affected by the pH of the tubular fluid. This is because the charged form of the drug (an organic acid in a high luminal pH environment or

Table 11.1
Drugs which are actively secreted by the proximal tubule

Organic acids	Organic bases
Penicillins	Amiloride
Cephalosporins	Quinidine
Sulphonamides	Tetracycline
Furosemide (frusemide)	
Thiazides	
Salicylates	
Probenicid	

Drugs and the kidney box 2

Follow-up on Mrs Johnson

The results of Mrs Johnson's blood tests come back, indicating that the serum digoxin level (taken some 8h after the last dose) is 3.9 nmol/L. This is well outside the recommended therapeutic range (0.6–2.3 nmol/L) and, taken in conjunction with her clinical features, is indicative of digoxin toxicity.

Furthermore, her plasma biochemistry results now show some further deterioration in renal function, with the urea being *12.1 mmol/L and the creatinine *0.16 mmol/L. These results suggest that her poor fluid intake (due to nausea), in addition to her vomiting, have led to plasma volume contraction with a fall in renal blood flow and hence in GFR. This worsening renal impairment in turn would have led to further digoxin accumulation, setting up a vicious cycle of deterioration in her condition. Apart from the unpleasant gastrointestinal features experienced by this patient, other toxic effects of digoxin include visual disturbances and cardiac arrhythmias. The latter may be quite serious and are exacerbated by low plasma potassium levels which may occur as a result of diuretic therapy and/or vomiting in this setting.

Fortunately, with temporary cessation of digoxin and restoration of her hydration state, Mrs Johnson's digoxin toxicity state subsided, and she was later stabilized on a smaller daily dose of the drug (0.0625 mg).

It is now worth reviewing some of the factors which led Mrs Johnson into so much trouble.

(*Values outside the normal range; see Appendix.)

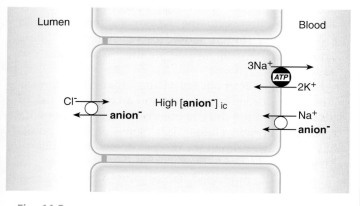

Fig. 11.3
Schematic of proximal tubular cell showing mechanism for transepithelial secretion of an organic acid (e.g. anionic drug).

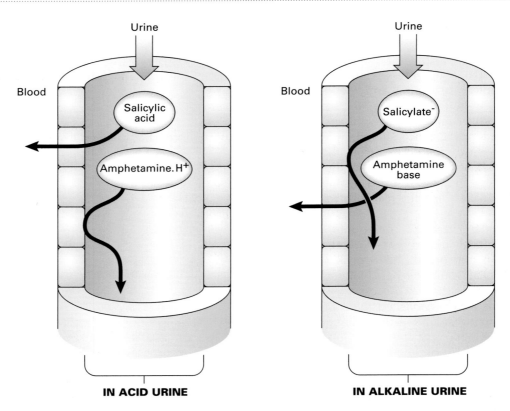

Fig. 11.4
Schematic of effect of altering urine pH on the excretion of acidic and basic drugs.

an organic base in a low luminal pH environment) is more water-soluble, favouring excretion (Fig. 11.4). Excretion of acidic drugs is therefore increased by raising the urinary pH, and the excretion of basic drugs is favoured by the excretion of an acidic urine. This may be important when facilitating drug excretion following overdosage, e.g. alkalinization of the urine with bicarbonate infusion to enhance aspirin excretion.

Finally, some drugs prevent the tubular secretion of other drugs by competing for binding to common transporters in the proximal tubule. This may be used therapeutically to enhance the desired effect of the drug and extend its half-life, e.g. treatment with the organic acid probenecid can cause an increase in serum penicillin concentrations and hence allow a reduced frequency of administration.

See box 2.

Drug dosing in renal failure

It is clear that Mrs Johnson had pre-existing renal impairment. Although her baseline serum creatinine was only just outside the normal range, it can be shown by using the Cockroft–Gault formula (see Chapter 5) that her GFR was considerably reduced, at around 29 mL/min, when she first presented to hospital. Thus the dose and/or dosage interval of drugs such as digoxin (that are very largely excreted by the kidney) should have been modified to avoid accumulation and the attendant risk of toxicity. This risk should be considered before the administration of any drug to a patient with renal impairment, and any adverse reaction occurring in temporal relationship to a drug being started should be considered as being caused by the drug unless another explanation can be found.

Several characteristics of a drug suggest that there is a need for dosage adjustment and an increased risk of toxicity when the drug is prescribed for patients with renal impairment (Table 11.2). Some of these points have already arisen in the discussion about the case of Mrs Johnson.

Numerous published tables and algorithms are available to guide the therapeutic use of a wide variety of drugs in patients with different degrees of renal failure. Some examples are given in this chapter but further details can be obtained from reference texts.

PART B

Renal impairment induced by drugs

Drugs and the kidney box 3

A predictable reaction

Roger Woodruffe is a 60-year-old man who presents with recent pain in his left knee joint that has limited his golfing activities. He has a history of hypertension, well controlled on a combination of an angiotensin-converting enzyme (ACE) inhibitor (perindopril 4 mg/day) and a loop diuretic (furosemide [frusemide] 40 mg/day). He is otherwise well. His blood pressure at the time he is seen is 145/95 mmHg. His serum biochemistry was last measured 6 months ago with the following results:

Sodium 140 mmol/L
Potassium 5.0 mmol/L
Chloride 105 mmol/L
Bicarbonate 23 mmol/L
*Urea 12.1 mmol/L
*Creatinine 0.16 mmol/L.

His doctor prescribes a non-steroidal anti-inflammatory drug (NSAID), diclofenac, 50 mg twice daily.

Mr Woodruffe returns for review in 10 days complaining of ankle swelling and mild dyspnoea on exertion. His blood pressure is now 175/105 mmHg and he has pitting oedema bilaterally. His doctor orders a new serum biochemical profile which shows the creatinine has risen to *0.24 mmol/L and the potassium is now elevated at *6.6 mmol/L. The serum albumin is normal at 41 g/L. Urinalysis shows only a trace of protein, and a midstream urine specimen reveals no increased excretion of cells and no bacterial growth. A full blood count is normal, with no increased eosinophil count to suggest that an allergic reaction is involved.

This case raises the issues associated with prescribing drugs with predictable effects on renal haemodynamics and transport for patients with already impaired renal function. By understanding the relevant physiology and pharmacology, it will become clear that Mr Woodruffe was at high risk of renal functional deterioration from the prescription of the NSAID diclofenac.

(*Values outside the normal range; see Appendix.)

Table 11.2
Characteristics of drugs that predict that a dosage adjustment should be made in renal disease

1. **Primary urinary excretion of the parent drug or metabolites**
   In general, if greater than 50% of a drug or its active metabolites is normally excreted in the urine, a dosage reduction will be necessary to prevent accumulation and potential toxicity (e.g. gentamicin, allopurinol).
2. **Low therapeutic index**
   Because of a narrow therapeutic range of efficacy of the drug, accumulation will result in significant toxicity (e.g. digoxin).
3. **High protein binding**
   Accumulation of organic acids in chronic renal failure will displace acidic drugs from albumin and increase free drug in the plasma, so that the target therapeutic concentration range (measuring total drug) should be adjusted downwards (e.g. phenytoin).
4. **A small volume of distribution of the drug**
   Changes in body water that occur in renal disease are more likely to impact on drugs that are distributed in smaller volumes (e.g. highly protein-bound drugs).

Renal actions of non-steroidal anti-inflammatory drugs

NSAIDs inhibit the formation of prostaglandins through the inhibition of cyclo-oxygenase (COX). Prostaglandins have a vasodilatory effect in the kidney, which is of particular significance in the presence of renal impairment. In this situation, glomerular filtration is maintained by increasing renal blood flow through afferent arteriolar vasodilatation (mediated by prostaglandins) and efferent arteriolar vasoconstriction (mediated by angiotensin II). Blockade of these compensatory mechanisms to maintain renal blood flow and GFR will be reflected by an increase in serum creatinine. Thus, prescription of NSAIDs in the presence of pre-existing renal impairment will commonly aggravate the degree of renal failure. This effect is exacerbated by concomitant use of ACE inhibitors and diuretics, which will further reduce the glomerular pressure and thus the driving force for glomerular filtration (see Chapter 5).

As prostaglandins also promote natriuresis by interfering with tubular sodium reabsorption, and blunt the effects of antidiuretic hormone on the tubular reabsorption of water, inhibition of prostaglandin production by NSAIDs results in salt and water retention, with resultant hypertension and oedema. Inhibition of prostaglandin synthesis also secondarily inhibits renin release, causing hyporeninaemic hypoaldosteronism which results in the impairment of distal tubular potassium secretion and hence hyperkalaemia. As these effects are caused by alterations in 'normal' physiological function, the urinalysis is unremarkable (minimal proteinuria or haematuria) and the urinary sediment is bland. In general, the abnormalities are corrected by withdrawal of the NSAID and any additional drugs affecting plasma volume and glomerular haemodynamics.

In summary, it is likely that all of Mr Woodruffe's problems at his second presentation – the worsening of renal function and hypertension, fluid retention and hyperkalaemia – are caused by the inhibition of renal COX by the NSAID diclofenac.

COX exists in two isoforms. COX 1 is constitutively expressed in the kidney and gastrointestinal tract, while COX 2 is expressed in inflamed tissues. Recently, drugs which selectively inhibit COX 2 have been developed for use in inflammatory conditions with the expectation that the side effect profile will be better than for the previously available non-selective COX 1 and 2 inhibitors. However, experience to date suggests that, while gastrointestinal side effects with the selective COX 2 inhibitors are greatly reduced, the effects on renal function and electrolyte homeostasis are comparable to the non-selective agents.

Drugs and the kidney box 4

Course and outcome

Mr Woodruffe is advised to cease the diclofenac, furosemide (frusemide) and perindopril, and is changed to sustained-release verapamil 240 mg/day as a replacement antihypertensive.

After 1 week, his oedema has largely resolved, the blood pressure has improved to 150/90 and his serum creatinine has fallen to *0.17 mmol/L, with normal electrolytes.

(*Values outside the normal range; see Appendix.)

Mechanisms of nephrotoxicity

It is clear from the above case that drug-induced nephrotoxicity may be mediated by alterations in renal haemodynamics via an effect on humoral systems within the kidney. However, drugs may also be directly nephrotoxic to renal cells (largely affecting the tubular cells) or cause immunologically mediated damage. Thus a drug may directly induce acute tubular necrosis (although haemodynamic influences may also be involved), or trigger interstitial nephritis or, occasionally, glomerular injury.

Both of these latter mechanisms may be invoked in different patients in the nephrotoxicity observed

with NSAIDs, in addition to the physiologically predictable haemodynamic and tubular transport effects noted above. In particular, NSAID-induced interstitial nephritis is seen relatively commonly, partly because of the high prevalence of usage in the community.

Drug-induced interstitial nephritis

Idiosyncratic responses to many drugs may include an acute interstitial nephritis. Because of the inflammatory nature of the condition, characterized by an interstitial inflammatory response with eosinophilic infiltration (Fig. 11.5), the urinalysis will generally show haematuria and proteinuria and often granular casts on urine microscopy. Renal function will generally deteriorate because of interstitial inflammation and oedema, causing a reduction in renal blood flow and GFR. The inflammatory cell infiltrate consists of a variety of cells, including B and T lymphocytes, plasma cells, natural killer cells and macrophages. In the majority of instances where T cell subsets have been studied in drug-induced interstitial nephritis, the CD4+ population predominates. Peripheral eosinophilia is often present and, in occasional cases, a more systemic 'allergic' response will result in skin rashes and arthralgia. NSAIDs have been well documented to cause interstitial nephritis up to 6 months after stable therapy. However, in Mr Woodruffe's case, the diagnosis of interstitial nephritis is not supported, as the urinalysis and urine sediment were not abnormal and systemic features were not prominent.

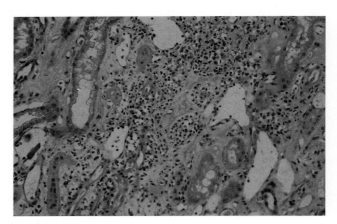

Fig. 11.5
Micrograph (stained with haematoxylin and eosin) showing acute interstitial nephritis. Note the intense inflammatory infiltrate and oedema in the interstitium; numerous eosinophils can be detected under high power.

Many drugs have been implicated as a cause of acute interstitial nephritis (Table 11.3), which can arise within a variable period from commencement of the drug. Thus, a deterioration in renal function in this setting should alert the clinician to the possibility of this diagnosis.

An improvement in renal function will generally follow the withdrawal of the offending agent. The time to recovery may vary from days to months. Renal biopsy is usually performed to confirm the diagnosis where there is severe renal impairment, or because of systemic features which raise the question of **vasculitis**. In these cases, short-term treatment with corticosteroids may be of benefit in shortening the natural course of the illness. Although in the majority of cases GFR returns to baseline values, there is a loss of functional renal tissue in many cases, characterized histologically by interstitial fibrosis and sometimes glomerulosclerosis. Factors associated with a greater loss of renal functional capacity include more severe initial renal failure, a slower rate of recovery after withdrawal of the offending agent, greater histological damage, older age group and lack of initial steroid therapy.

Drug-induced glomerular pathology

Glomerular pathology is less common than tubulo-interstitial injury in drug-induced nephrotoxicity. In general, glomerular damage presents as proteinuria and the most frequently observed pathology is membranous nephropathy. The frequency with which glomerular injury occurs in patients treated with certain drugs, notably gold and penicillamine (used mainly in rheumatoid arthritis), is high enough to warrant routine surveillance by urinalysis. In general, the prognosis of the glomerular lesion is favourable after withdrawal of the drug, with an improvement in proteinuria generally observed. The occurrence of **glomerulopathy** in this setting is not clearly dose-related, and the aetiology remains unclear.

NSAIDs may also induce a glomerulopathy, with minimal change nephropathy being the most widely recognized pathological lesion. However, this is rare, and is unlikely to be implicated in the deteriorating renal function in the case reviewed in the current chapter, as proteinuria was not present on urinalysis.

Important causes of nephrotoxicity

In the case of some drugs, nephrotoxicity may be dose-related and predictable, while in other cases the condition is an uncommon side effect, but may be frequently observed if there is a high usage of the particular agent in the community. Some examples of common or important causes of nephrotoxicity are discussed below.

Gentamicin

Gentamicin (and other aminoglycosides) require specific mention because of the serious and avoidable nature of the toxicity associated with this class of antibiotics. Aminoglycosides are almost entirely excreted by the kidney. Thus, in renal failure excretion of the drug is reduced and, unless dosage modification is made, toxicity is likely to occur, affecting both the kidney and inner ear. The effectiveness of an aminoglycoside in killing bacteria correlates with its peak concentration rather than with its steady state concentration, whereas the nephrotoxicity correlates with the steady state accumulation of the drug into proximal tubular cells. Thus, in renal failure the drug dosage remains the same but the dose interval should be increased. In patients with end-stage renal failure, where the only clearance is through the dialysis process, the dose interval may be up to every 3 days. This contrasts with agents such as digoxin (and cyclosporin, discussed below) where a therapeutic effect requires a defined steady state concentration to be maintained. In these cases the dose is reduced but the dosage interval remains constant.

In patients with any degree of renal impairment, the clearance of a renally excreted drug may be hard to predict. Thus, whenever accumulation of a drug poses a predictable risk of toxicity, serum concentrations of the drug just before the next scheduled dose (trough level) should be used to guide either the dose or the dosage interval, as appropriate.

Table 11.3
Drugs frequently implicated in acute interstitial nephritis

Antibiotics	Others
Penicillins (especially methicillin)	Phenytoin
Cephalosporins	Allopurinol
Sulphonamides	Aspirin
Rifampicin	Methyldopa
Quinolones	Carbamazepine
	Valproic acid
Diuretics	Diazepam
Thiazides	Interferon
Furosemide (frusemide)	Beta-blockers
	Quinine
NSAIDs	Doxepin
	Azathioprine

Cyclosporin

Cyclosporin A is an immunosuppressive drug which is largely metabolized in the liver, but the main clinical manifestation of toxicity is renal injury. Several mechanisms of toxicity are recognized. Cyclosporin A induces marked intrarenal vasoconstriction and a fall in GFR, with acute damage to the proximal tubules and ischaemic nephropathy in the longer term. A classic histological appearance of 'striped fibrosis' occurs in chronic cyclosporin nephrotoxicity. An **arteriopathy** is also well recognized with a syndrome consistent with haemolytic uraemic syndrome, characterized by activation of the coagulation system and intravascular haemolysis, resulting in anaemia, **thrombocytopenia** and impaired renal function.

As cyclosporin A is metabolized by the cytochrome-dependent mixed function oxidases in the liver, drugs which interact with this system may impair its metabolism, thus precipitating significant toxicity or, alternatively, accelerate metabolism resulting in loss of the immunosuppressive effect. As cyclosporin is widely used in renal transplantation, drug levels are closely monitored as fluctuations in renal function in this circumstance are common and a high cyclosporin level may provide evidence suggesting the development of nephrotoxicity.

Renal disease induced by non-prescription medicines

Epidemiological studies have clearly identified the ingestion of aspirin, phenacetin and caffeine in over-the-counter compound analgesic medications as a cause of a characteristic interstitial nephritis with **papillary necrosis**, associated with an increased propensity to uroepithelial carcinoma. This clinical entity of *analgesic nephropathy* has been the most prevalent clearly recognized cause of drug-induced end-stage renal failure within defined demographic populations (including Australia). Although analgesic nephropathy accounted for up to 22% of patients entering dialysis programs in the early 1980s, its incidence has steadily declined since the withdrawal of these med-

ications in combination form from over-the-counter sale. Long-term ingestion of NSAIDs has been implicated in the pathogenesis of some cases of interstitial nephritis and papillary necrosis. However, the incidence is relatively low compared with the former usage of the compound agents.

'Natural' therapies are increasingly being used for a variety of conditions in both western and eastern cultures. The constituents of such therapies are often poorly documented, and they may result in either dose-dependent or idiosyncratic side effects. One recently reported form of so-called 'Chinese Herb Nephropathy' related to the use of *Aristolochia frangchi* for weight reduction. This has been causally demonstrated to induce a rapidly progressive non-inflammatory interstitial fibrosis in the kidney, resulting in end-stage renal failure. Follow-up investigations in these patients have revealed an increased risk of uroepithelial cancer, high enough to justify recommendation of prophylactic nephrectomy before consideration of transplantation and immunosuppression.

Contrast agents

Intravenous administration of iodinated radiological contrast agents has been reported to be nephrotoxic, particularly in patients with volume depletion, pre-existing renal disease, diabetes mellitus or multiple myeloma. In general, an acute reversible decline in renal function is observed and, in severe cases, the underlying pathological lesion is acute tubular necrosis. The newer non-ionic compounds have been reported to be less nephrotoxic and are preferred, particularly in high-risk patients. It is recommended that intravenous saline loading be undertaken in these patients before the procedure, since this measure has been found to be protective in laboratory and clinical studies. Furthermore, agents that may exacerbate renal haemodynamic injury, such as NSAIDs and ACE inhibitors, should be ceased. In many instances, alternative means of imaging can now be undertaken, and these should be carefully considered in patients with advanced renal disease.

Self-assessment case study

A 68-year-old man with diet-controlled non-insulin-dependent diabetes develops hypotension and fever 16 h after the removal of an obstructing renal calculus using an endoscopic approach. The last serum creatinine available 1 month previously is 0.13 mmol/L, with a urea of 6.8 mmol/L and a serum potassium of 5.2 mmol/L. His past history includes mild–moderate cardiac failure treated with a combination of captopril and spironolactone. Doses of both of these drugs have been lowered recently because of hyperkalaemia. His additional medical problems include arthritis of both knees for which he takes regular non-steroidal anti-inflammatory drugs (NSAIDs). In an attempt to control his arthritis, he has recently lost a significant amount of weight and now weighs 62 kg.

Because of the risk of Gram-negative sepsis following urological intervention, treatment with gentamicin is recommended. He is commenced on 240 mg by intravenous injection (IVI) daily.

After studying this chapter you should be able to answer the following questions:

① What factors indicate that this man is likely to develop gentamicin nephrotoxicity?

② What factors should guide the prescription dosing schedule of gentamicin?

③ List this patients's comorbidity and drug use which predispose him to hyperkalaemia.

④ Briefly indicate the mechanisms whereby drugs may result in acute renal failure.

Answers see page 151

Self-assessment questions

① Define the elimination half-life of a drug and explain how this may be altered in renal impairment.

② What factors determine whether a drug is excreted by the kidney?

③ Describe the clinical and laboratory findings that differentiate an interstitial nephritis from a haemodynamic-mediated reduction in renal function.

Answers see page 151

ANSWERS

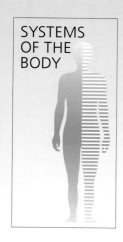

Chapter 1
Self-assessment case study answers

① What are the key clinical features suggestive of underlying urinary tract abnormality in this case?

The clinical features suggestive of an underlying urinary tract abnormality are:

- *Kidney infection in childhood (and any urinary infection in men or in women who are not sexually active) can suggest the presence of underlying abnormalities in the structure or function of the urinary tract.*
- *Asymptomatic bacteriuria and subsequent failure to eradicate infection suggests abnormalities in the drainage of the urinary tract. Although this may occur in normal pregnancy, it does not usually result in bacteriuria or infection.*
- *Nocturia can occur because of failure to empty the urinary bladder adequately (e.g. as occurs in reflux nephropathy), or because of damage to the distal tubules of the kidney resulting in failure to concentrate the urine (see Chapters 2 and 3). This results in an increased volume of urine, often manifesting as enuresis in children and nocturia in adults.*
- *As structural abnormalities of the kidney are often familial, the presence of symptoms suggestive of a similar problem in her siblings increases the likelihood of an anatomical defect being found.*
- *The presence of hypertension suggests renal parenchymal disease may be present.*

② What tests would have been done to confirm infection in this young woman?

Infection would initially be suggested by the finding of blood, protein, nitrites and leucocytes in the urine on urinalysis. An increased white cell excretion normally occurs in pregnancy, and there is also a marginal increase in normal urinary protein excretion. However, the additional abnormalities do not occur unless infection is present. Urine microscopy would have demonstrated bacteria and red and white cells. Over 10^5 bacteria, which cause a 'pure growth' on urine culture, are normally present in clinically significant infection. However, even smaller numbers of bacteria, when in a pure growth, may be significant.

③ Is it likely that she currently has a lower or upper urinary tract infection? What factors predispose her to developing a complicated (or upper urinary tract) infection?

She is likely to have lower urinary tract infection as dysuria and frequency are bladder and urethral symptoms, and her tenderness localizes to the bladder. Classic features of upper urinary infection – fever, loin tenderness and being generally 'unwell' – are not present. Lower urinary tract infection is more likely to develop into upper urinary infection in pregnancy because of incomplete bladder emptying and/or partial obstruction of the urinary tract caused by the uterus encroaching on the bladder. Ureteric contraction resulting in pooling of the urine in a dilated urinary tract also occurs in normal pregnancy. The presence of a horseshoe kidney is an additional factor resulting in impaired urinary drainage. Asymptomatic bacteriuria and recurrent infection increases the risk of ascending infection as this may be present without necessarily

causing symptoms; pyelonephritis may be an initial symptom.

④ What recommendations would you make about her current treatment and what follow-up investigations would you perform after the delivery of her child?

Because of recurrent infection and the risk of pyelonephritis in pregnancy, which may increase uterine irritability and precipitate premature labour, prophylactic antibiotics should be prescribed. After the urine is rendered sterile with a full 2-week course of oral antibiotics, a single night-time dose of either a cephalosporin or amoxicillin (both of which are safe for the developing fetus) should be administered until after delivery. Routine urine culture is recommended on a monthly basis and, if breakthrough infection occurs, a full course of antibiotics, determined by the sensitivity of the organisms and the safety of the fetus, should be prescribed. Blood pressure should be treated as she is at high risk for pre-eclampsia (exacerbation of hypertension) later in pregnancy. After delivery, her baby should be screened for abnormalities of the urinary tract, and she should be warned that, if her baby has an unexplained febrile illness, urine infection should be considered. She should have further renal imaging, but not sooner than 3 months after delivery. If imaging is performed before this time, dilatation of the urinary tract owing to pregnancy rather than because of intrinsic renal disease may complicate the interpretation.

Self-assessment question answers

① Can you describe the major anatomical components of the urinary tract?

The major anatomical components of the urinary tract are two kidneys, two ureters, bladder and urethra. Renal artery, veins, nerves and the ureter enter (and/or leave) the kidney through the hilum.

② Describe the embryological derivation of the major structures of the kidney.

The glomeruli and initial parts of the kidney tubule are largely derived from the metanephros. The collecting ducts, derived from the ureteric bud, invade the developing metanephros to form a functional kidney. The metanephros also forms the additional components of the kidney, i.e. the mesangial cells which support the glomerular capillaries, endothelial cells, smooth muscle cells and matrix components.

③ Describe the mechanisms that normally protect the urinary tract from infection.

Urinary infection is normally prevented by the continuous unobstructed flow of urine, and a hostile biochemical environment, i.e. high osmolarity, acidic pH and high urea concentration. Local host defences also include white cells within the bladder mucosa and prostatic secretions that have bactericidal properties.

④ What are the principles of treatment of uncomplicated lower urinary tract infection and upper urinary tract infection?

In lower urinary tract infection, a precipitating cause should be sought (e.g. contraceptive diaphragm use, altered sexual activity) and appropriate advice given. A high fluid intake is recommended and a short course of antibiotics (3 days) is generally sufficient to eradicate infection. Dysuria may be alleviated by alkalinization of the urine with a bicarbonate-based medication in tablet or solution.

Upper urinary tract infection often requires analgesia, intravenous fluids, and appropriate antibiotic treatment (5 days IV and subsequent oral treatment) for 2 weeks. Imaging of the urinary tract is generally indicated after treatment of an acute infection.

Chapter 2
Self-assessment case study answers

① What features of the history and examination are suggestive of hypovolaemia?

The tiredness and dizziness are consistent with a state of low blood pressure related to hypovolaemia. On examination, the dry mouth and low blood pressure with postural drop are also suggestive of a low volume state, as is the resting tachycardia.

② Although no drugs have been formally prescribed, what medication might the patient be taking of her own accord?

Either a loop diuretic (e.g. furosemide; frusemide) or an early distal acting diuretic (e.g. a thiazide), could produce this clinical and electrolyte pattern. Similar results could also be produced by taking a purgative, although the urine sodium concentration would be expected to be low.

③ What biochemical analysis would help distinguish between furosemide (frusemide) and thiazide use?

The urine calcium excretion would be normal or high with furosemide (frusemide) use, but low during thiazide use.

④ How would surreptitious diuretic use best be excluded?

A biochemical screen of the urine for various chemical classes of drugs should detect active use and excretion of one of these agents.

⑤ In this patient, the urine calcium excretion was found to be very low, and no drugs were detected in the urine. In which segment of the nephron would you predict that there was an inherited or acquired functional defect?

The early distal (convoluted) tubule. This inherited disorder is known as Gitelman's syndrome and is caused by a faulty NaCl cotransport molecule in the early distal tubule cells. In addition to the features described here, hypomagnesaemia caused by urinary magnesium wasting is also seen in this condition.

Self-assessment question answers

① List three features on physical examination suggestive of hypervolaemia (volume expansion).

Peripheral oedema, elevated jugular venous pressure, crepitations at the lung bases, recent gain in weight and, in some circumstances, hypertension.

② Indicate the expected change from normal in each of the following parameters during hypervolaemia: plasma renin, plasma aldosterone, plasma atrial natriuretic peptide, glomerular filtration rate.

Renin is decreased, aldosterone is decreased, atrial natriuretic peptide is increased, glomerular filtration rate is increased (unless there is renal disease).

③ What changes would you expect in the plasma potassium concentration and urinary excretion of potassium during prolonged treatment with high dose spironolactone?

Plasma potassium may rise and urinary potassium excretion would be reduced, as a consequence of interference by spironolactone with the action of aldosterone on the cortical collecting duct.

④ A 500-mL transfusion of whole blood is given to a patient with shock. The transfused blood has a haematocrit (packed cell volume) of 42%. Immediately after transfusion, what is the change in total intracellular fluid volume and extracellular fluid volume in the patient?

The transfused blood will add 210 mL of intracellular fluid in the form of red blood cells, and 290 mL to the extracellular fluid in the form of plasma. In some circumstances, redistribution of these volumes may occur after transfusion.

Chapter 3
Self-assessment case study answers

① Does this patient show inappropriate failure to concentrate the urine or inappropriate failure to dilute the urine?

Since the plasma is markedly hypotonic, and since the osmotic control mechanisms should respond by diluting the urine to excrete some of the excess water retained in the extracellular fluid, the fact that the urine osmolality is relatively high suggests that a failure to dilute the urine appropriately has developed.

② What laboratory evidence confirms the clinical impression that he is not hypovolaemic?

The relatively high urine sodium concentration suggests that there has not been activation of sodium-conserving mechanisms which would be expected in the presence of significant hypovolaemia.

③ What influences might be acting to determine the plasma level of antidiuretic hormone (ADH) in this clinical setting?

While the hypotonicity of the plasma in itself would be expected to inhibit ADH release, the patient has suffered stress and is in pain, both of which act as non-osmotic stimuli to the release of ADH. Furthermore, the injuries affecting his lung and brain may also act as triggers for central release of ADH, which in this circumstance is 'inappropriate' to the low plasma osmolality and normal circulating blood volume. This scenario is typical of the acute development of a syndrome of inappropriate ADH secretion (SIADH).

④ What management would you suggest for the hyponatraemia in this context?

Attention must be given to the cause of his likely high ADH level: thus appropriate relief of pain and correct management of his lung and cerebral injuries should gradually cause this to subside. In the meantime,

145

moderate restriction of free water intake (both orally and by avoiding electrolyte-free intravenous fluids) should be sufficient to prevent the plasma sodium falling further.

Self-assessment question answers

① What properties of the loop of Henle are critical to its operation as a countercurrent multiplication system?
The relevant properties of the loop of Henle are:

- *its hairpin configuration*
- *the existence of an active solute pump capable of generating an osmolality gradient between the lumen of the thick ascending limb and the adjacent interstitium*
- *the water impermeability of the ascending limb*
- *the high water permeability of the descending limb.*

② What changes in which parameters of the loop of Henle function would be expected to decrease its capacity to generate a hypertonic medullary interstitium?
The concentrating power of the loop would be decreased by:

- *a reduction in the activity of the solute pump in the walls of the thick ascending limb*
- *an increase in flow rate through the loop*
- *interference with the water impermeability of the ascending limb.*

Another factor which is not variable in a given kidney is a reduction in the length of the loop.

③ Name, in order, the physiological changes which occur after ingestion of a large volume of water leading to its excretion shortly afterwards through the kidney.
Following ingestion of a large volume of water, the following sequence of changes occurs: rapid absorption of water through the upper gastrointestinal tract → slight dilution of the plasma → detection of reduced plasma osmolality by hypothalamic osmoreceptors → simultaneous suppression of thirst and suppression of ADH release from the hypothalamus via its axonal processes in the posterior pituitary → reduced water permeability of the collecting ducts in the kidney → excretion of maximally dilute urine.

④ Name the sequence of cellular actions which follow binding of antidiuretic hormone (ADH) to its receptor in the collecting duct of the kidney.
The following sequence occurs after binding of ADH (arginine vasopressin) to the V2 receptor on the basolateral membrane of renal collecting duct cells: activation of receptor-coupled G protein → activation of membrane-bound adenyl cyclase → generation of increased intracellular levels of cyclic AMP → activation of phosphokinases → mobilization by cytoskeletal elements of preformed intracytoplasmic vesicles containing aquaporin 2 water channels → insertion of aquaporin 2 channels into the apical membrane of collecting duct cells → increased flux of water from the lumen through the apical membrane and hence through the cell and the basolateral membrane into the blood.

Chapter 4
Self-assessment case study answers

① What is the overall pattern of acid–base disturbance in this patient?
Metabolic acidosis, with incomplete respiratory compensation.

② What is the anion gap in this patient?
The anion gap is $(135 + 5.2) − (97 + 14) = 29.2\,mmol/L$. This is higher than the normal range ($12–18\,mmol/L$), suggesting that the acidosis can be attributed to the appearance of a 'new' acid anion.

③ What is the likely cause of the disturbance in this case?
In view of the patient's poor cardiac output, poor peripheral perfusion and ischaemic leg, it is likely that considerable anaerobic metabolism is occurring in the tissues, with a generation of lactic acid as the endpoint. Thus, lactate is likely to be the unmeasured anion expanding the anion gap.

④ What would you expect the urine pH to be?
Given that renal function is not greatly impaired and that there is a significant systemic acidosis, over a period of days the kidney would increase its capacity for acid excretion, including the generation of increased amounts of ammonia with which acid is excreted as ammonium ions. The urine pH would be expected to fall below 6.0.

⑤ What are the principles of treatment?
Reversing the cause of the poor tissue perfusion would be a primary goal, and this would involve optimum management of his heart failure, as well as removal or dissolution of his femoral artery embolus which would hopefully reverse the hypoxic conditions in his tissues. Provision of adequate oxygen supplementation in his inspired air would assist in this. Treatment of the acidosis itself is generally recommended only where the pH remains below 7.25 because of inadequate compensation. This may involve oral or intravenous supplementation with sodium bicarbonate.

⑥ What would the effect of a bicarbonate infusion be on his plasma potassium concentration?
The plasma potassium would fall if bicarbonate is infused to correct the acidosis since extracellular acidosis promotes potassium movement out of cells, and this is reversed by raising the extracellular pH.

Self-assessment question answers

① What would the effect on systemic acid–base balance be if a patient were given long-term treatment with a carbonic anhydrase inhibitor such as acetazolamide?
Acetazolamide interferes with the ability of the proximal tubule to reabsorb bicarbonate ions, which depends on the enzyme carbonic anhydrase acting both within proximal tubular cells and in the proximal tubular lumen. Blockade of this enzyme by acetazolamide leads to bicarbonate wasting and a degree of systemic metabolic acidosis of the normal anion gap type.

② Where in the nephron is the steepest gradient of pH between the plasma and the luminal fluid?

Acidification of the luminal fluid against a steep hydrogen ion concentration gradient occurs chiefly in the most distal nephron segments, particularly the outer medullary collecting duct where acid-secreting pumps are abundant in the apical cell membrane of the tubular epithelial cells, and the epithelium has a low hydrogen ion permeability, allowing maintenance of the steep transtubular pH gradient.

③ Name three changes in the plasma which stimulate an increase in hydrogen ion secretion by the nephron.

A decreased plasma pH, an increased blood pCO_2 and hypokalaemia all stimulate tubular acid secretion. Note that increased circulating levels of aldosterone also enhance hydrogen ion secretion in the distal nephron.

④ Give three causes of a metabolic acidosis with a normal anion gap.

Infusion or ingestion of hydrochloric acid, diarrhoea or equivalent lower gastrointestinal loss, and failure of renal tubular mechanisms to reabsorb bicarbonate or secrete hydrogen ions (renal tubular acidosis) all cause metabolic acidosis with a normal anion gap.

⑤ Name three factors which perpetuate the systemic alkalosis which follows prolonged vomiting.

In addition to the initiation of alkalosis because of loss of gastric acid, there is stimulation of proximal bicarbonate reabsorption due to the hypovolaemia which follows gastric losses of sodium and water. This hypovolaemia also triggers aldosterone release which enhances distal acid secretion and perpetuates the systemic alkalosis. Finally, potassium is also lost in the vomitus, and is excreted by the kidney because of high circulating aldosterone levels. Hypokalaemia promotes tubular acid secretion and renal ammonia synthesis, again amplifying the systemic alkalosis.

Chapter 5
Self-assessment case study answers

① What are the factors involved in the development of this man's acute renal failure?

His acute renal failure can be explained by poor renal perfusion because of prolonged systemic hypotension, and likely rhabdomyolysis with myoglobin released from damaged muscle causing direct tubular toxicity. The increased serum potassium, disproportionate to the elevation in serum urea and creatinine, suggests that there is net addition of potassium to the extracellular fluid, as well as a reduction in urinary potassium excretion caused by the renal failure. Oliguria and dark urine also support this diagnosis, but this is non-specific and may occur with acute renal failure of any cause.

② What additional biochemical abnormalities are likely to be present?

As rhabdomyolysis is suspected, an increased plasma creatine phosphokinase would be expected. As damaged muscle cells release their intracellular content into the circulation, an increased plasma phosphate is expected. As this phosphate precipitates with calcium, plasma calcium falls but ionized calcium is normal. Urine will contain myoglobin, which crossreacts with haemoglobin

on urinalysis, but haematuria can be excluded by examination of the urine sediment where heavily pigmented casts, but no red cells, are observed.

③ Describe the immediate treatment of his acute renal failure.

His most immediate problem is hyperkalaemia with its potential to cause lethal cardiac arrhythmias. Initial management includes establishment of secure intravenous access with rapid administration of intravenous normal saline. Intravenous calcium gluconate should be given to stabilize the membrane potential in the cardiac conducting tissue. This is followed by sodium bicarbonate (in different IV lines, or at least after flushing the calcium from the line to avoid calcium carbonate precipitation), intravenous glucose and intravenous or subcutaneous insulin and nebulized Ventolin, all of which promote a shift of potassium into cells. Fluids should be given until his hypovolaemia is corrected, and if urine flow is not subsequently established, diuretics may be given. Once urine flow is established, alkalinization of the urine using intravenous sodium bicarbonate reduces the tubular toxicity of myoglobin. If oliguria persists, dialysis may be necessary.

④ Describe in general terms the expected course and prognosis of his renal failure.

Rhabdomyolysis generally has a good prognosis, although dialysis may initially be required. During the recovery from acute tubular necrosis, polyuria and increased urinary electrolyte losses occur, necessitating vigorous replacement therapy. However, recovery of renal function is usually complete.

Self-assessment question answers

① Describe the factors involved in determining glomerular filtration.

Glomerular filtration rate (GFR) depends on the following factors:

- *Glomerular capillary pressure which 'drives' filtration. This is largely determined by systemic blood pressure, renal blood flow and afferent and efferent arteriolar tone.*
- *Plasma oncotic pressure, which tends to keep fluid in the capillaries and inhibit filtration. This is largely determined by plasma proteins.*
- *Tubular pressure, which is normally low in the absence of tubular obstruction, and thus favours filtration from the capillary into Bowman's space and hence to the tubule.*
- *Glomerular capillary surface area: in effect, if less functioning kidney tissue is present, less filtration occurs.*

② Define the renal clearance of a substance and explain why clearance of creatinine reflects kidney function.

The clearance of a substance is defined as the apparent volume of plasma that is completely cleared of a substance in a defined unit of time. If a substance is not significantly secreted or reabsorbed by the tubules of the kidney, then its clearance reflects the GFR (see Fig. 5.5). Creatinine is largely excreted by glomerular filtration. However, a small proportion is secreted by the tubules of the kidney. Thus, creatinine clearance slightly overestimates GFR. This overestimation becomes more

147

significant when renal function is impaired and tubular secretion accounts for an increased proportion of creatinine clearance.

③ What are the clinical and laboratory features that differentiate physiological oliguria from acute tubular necrosis?

Physiological oliguria is characterized by a low urine output in the presence of reduced renal perfusion. Thus clinical features of hypotension and/or dehydration are often present. Evidence of intact tubular function is present in physiological dehydration, i.e. the ability to concentrate urine and reduce renal sodium excretion is characteristic of reversible oliguria. Thus, a high urine osmolality and low urine sodium are expected. As urea may be reabsorbed by the tubule if urine flow rate is reduced and creatinine may be secreted by the tubule, a high plasma urea : creatinine ratio reflects poor renal perfusion and intact tubular function.

In acute tubular necrosis, the ability to concentrate urine and reabsorb sodium is impaired. Thus a low urinary osmolality and high urine sodium occurs.

Chapter 6
Self-assessment case study answers

① What is the most likely clinical diagnosis?

In the absence of hepatic and cardiac disease, the most likely diagnosis is nephrotic syndrome.

② Name two other features required to make this clinical diagnosis.

Proteinuria and hypoalbuminaemia.

③ Why has the patient developed oedema?

Urinary protein loss leads to hypoalbuminaemia. Peripheral oedema develops, partially due to hypoalbuminaemia and therefore low plasma oncotic pressure (so that excess oedema fluid leaks from the capillaries), and also because of renal sodium and water retention.

④ List at least three possible complications of this condition and the pathophysiological factors involved.

Deep venous thrombosis owing to hypercoagulability caused by increased hepatic synthesis of thrombotic factors and urinary loss of antithrombotic factors; hyperlipidaemia caused by increased hepatic synthesis of lipoproteins; increased risk of infection because of urinary loss of immunoglobulins and other defence proteins; chronic renal failure owing to natural progression of the disease.

⑤ In a patient of this age, what is the most likely renal histopathological diagnosis?

Membranous glomerulonephritis. There are a number of other possible diagnoses, including focal sclerosing glomerulonephritis and amyloidosis.

⑥ Describe the likely renal histopathological features.

Thickening of capillary loops on light microscopy; electron-dense deposits between the glomerular basement membrane and visceral glomerular epithelial cell on electron microscopy; IgG and C3 in a capillary wall distribution on immunofluorescence microscopy.

① List four factors which will favour the formation of oedema at the level of a capillary.

Increase in hydrostatic pressure within the capillary lumen, reduced concentration of plasma proteins causing reduced plasma oncotic pressure, increased leakiness of the capillary wall and reduced lymphatic flow.

② Which three structures comprise the glomerular capillary wall?

Glomerular endothelial cell, glomerular basement membrane and visceral glomerular epithelial cell.

③ What is the definition of nephrotic syndrome?

Heavy proteinuria causing hypoalbuminaemia and oedema.

④ List the principal complications of nephrotic syndrome and their pathophysiology.

Hypercholesterolaemia, thrombosis, infection, renal failure, malnutrition. See Table 6.3 for pathophysiology.

⑤ What pathological features are expected in the renal biopsy of a patient with minimal change disease?

Normal light and immunofluorescence microscopy, diffuse fusion of podocytes on electron microscopy.

Chapter 7
Self-assessment case study answers

① Explain how urinary examination would help to narrow the differential diagnosis in this case.

The presence of red blood cells (especially dysmorphic), casts and protein in the urine would all point to an upper urinary tract (i.e. renal parenchymal) origin for the bleeding; red blood cells without the other urinary abnormalities would point to a lower tract origin; positive dipstick for blood without red cells on microscopy would point to pigmenturia (i.e. haemoglobinuria or myoglobinuria).

② Based on the other clinical features, what is the most likely diagnosis?

The recurrent nature of the haematuria and sore throat occurring only a few days before presentation points to a diagnosis of mesangial IgA disease rather than post-streptococcal or postinfectious glomerulonephritis.

③ What other clinical features are required to make a diagnosis of 'the nephritic syndrome'? What is the pathogenesis of each feature?

The nephritic syndrome consists of macroscopic haematuria, elevated serum creatinine and hypertension. The haematuria is caused by the leakage of the red cells from the glomerulus into the tubular lumen. Hypertension is due to renal salt and water retention and in part to the release of vasoactive hormones. Reduced renal function is caused by structural damage (e.g. proliferation within the glomerulus, but also tubulointerstitial inflammation and scarring) as well as intrarenal haemodynamic changes because of vasoactive hormone release.

④ What are the main renal histopathological features of this disease?

Mesangial proliferation on light microscopy; mesangial electron-dense deposits on electron microscopy; IgA in mesangial distribution on immunofluorescence microscopy.

Self-assessment question answers

① What are the diagnostic clinical features of the acute nephritic syndrome? Describe their pathogenesis.
   Haematuria (because of leakage of blood cells across the glomerular capillary wall), hypertension (caused by salt and water retention and activation of the renin–angiotensin system), renal functional impairment (due to vasoactive hormone release and structural injury). See Table 6.2.

② List three conditions causing acute glomerulonephritis (GN) in which the serum concentration of complement components C3 or C3 and C4 may be reduced.
   Post-streptococcal GN, mesangiocapillary GN, systemic lupus erythematosus (SLE).

③ Which diagnostic serological tests are also involved in the immunopathogenesis of SLE, Wegener's granulomatosus, Goodpasture's syndrome, hepatitis B and C respectively?
   Anti-dsDNA antibody, ANCA, anti-GBM antibody, HBsAg, anti-HCV antibody, respectively.

④ Describe five clinical features which may be used to distinguish post-streptococcal GN from IgA disease.
   See Table 6.4.

⑤ List three ways in which antibodies may be associated with the glomerular basement membrane in acute GN.
   In situ immune complex formation, deposition of circulating immune complex, reaction with intrinsic glomerular antigen.

Chapter 8
Self-assessment case study answers

① What is the most likely explanation for nocturia?
   *The patient probably has diabetic nephropathy. Nocturia is most likely to be a symptom of chronic renal failure (because of impaired urinary concentrating ability and the necessity to excrete some of the obligate osmolar load – derived from her diet – at night time).
   Alternatively, the nocturia could be caused by osmotic diuresis because of poor control of her diabetes with glycosuria and ketonuria.*

② If she were to have had a renal biopsy 10 years previously, what would have been the likely histopathological features?
   Uniform thickening of the glomerular basement membrane and mesangial expansion. Concurrent with the development of chronic renal failure she would be expected to develop scarring in the glomerulus (glomerulosclerosis) and tubulointerstitial fibrosis.

③ Why are her ankle jerks absent?
   Because of peripheral neuropathy associated with both diabetes and chronic renal failure.

④ What is the explanation for her tender tibiae?
   Renal bone disease because of hyperparathyroidism and vitamin D deficiency.

⑤ The patient also complained of weakness, and conjunctival pallor was found. What is the likely explanation?
   Normochromic/normocytic anaemia because of erythropoietin deficiency.

Self-assessment question answers

① Which of the following features suggests chronic rather than acute renal failure?
   (a) Nocturia for several months
   (b) Anaemia
   (c) Small echogenic kidneys
   (d) Bone pain
   (e) Intact ankle jerks
   Nocturia for several months, anaemia, small echogenic kidneys, bone pain.

② List the following clinical features in order of their appearance as glomerular filtration rate falls in progressive chronic renal failure.
   (a) Oedema
   (b) Anaemia
   (c) Need for dialysis to sustain life
   (d) Asymptomatic bone disease.
   Asymptomatic bone disease, anaemia, oedema, need for dialysis to sustain life.

③ List the following causes of chronic renal failure according to their incidence in developed countries (most to least common):
   (a) analgesic nephropathy
   (b) diabetes mellitus
   (c) polycystic kidney disease
   (d) glomerulonephritis
   (e) hypertension.
   Glomerulonephritis, diabetes mellitus, hypertension, polycystic kidney disease, analgesic nephropathy.

④ List the major factors which lead to secondary hyperparathyroidism in chronic renal failure.
   Hyperphosphataemia because of inability to excrete phosphate; impaired vitamin D activation (because of hyperphosphataemia and renal parenchymal loss); increased secretion of parathyroid hormone because of low ionized calcium and low calcitriol levels; low ionized calcium levels caused by impaired intestinal calcium absorption (because of low calcitriol) and hyperphosphataemia.

Chapter 9
Self-assessment case study answers

① What possible cause of secondary hypertension is suggested by this story?
   A high mineralocorticoid secretion state (such as primary aldosteronism) is suggested by the combination of persistent hypokalaemia with hypertension. The relatively short history in a middle-aged patient also favours this secondary cause rather than essential hypertension. Other possible but less likely underlying causes include phaeochromocytoma or renal artery stenosis.

② What further investigation would you recommend?

Measurement of plasma renin and aldosterone levels may provide supportive evidence for primary hyperaldosteronism (Conn's syndrome). Ideally, these measurements should be made while the patient is not taking beta-blockers, which suppress renin production. Although ACE inhibitors normally reduce aldosterone levels and secondarily increase plasma renin, in the presence of an autonomous tumour or adrenal gland hyperplasia producing large amounts of aldosterone, a high plasma aldosterone:renin ratio would generally still be obtained even in the presence of ACE inhibitor therapy. A further dynamic challenge can be provided by resampling the blood for renin and aldosterone after a test dose of furosemide (frusemide) is given intravenously. The resulting hypovolaemic stimulus would normally prompt an increase in renin and aldosterone secretion, but the renin rise would be blunted or absent in the presence of an aldosterone-secreting adrenal neoplasm. It should be noted that more detailed endocrine testing and genetic analysis can be performed when specific types of mineralocorticoid overproduction are suspected.

③ What form of imaging may be helpful in defining an underlying adrenal neoplasm?

CT scanning of the abdomen with fine cuts through the adrenal glands may define a unilateral adrenocortical adenoma or bilateral adrenal hyperplasia.

④ If primary aldosteronism is confirmed, what are the treatment options?

If a unilateral adenoma is defined and is proven by adrenal venous sampling to be the source of autonomous aldosterone overproduction, surgery to remove the adrenal gland (by open surgery or laparoscopy) can provide a definitive form of treatment. In some patients with adenomas and in the majority in whom bilateral adrenal hyperplasia is defined, blockade of the renal action of aldosterone using the receptor antagonist spironolactone can produce acceptable long-term control of hypertension and correction of hypokalaemia.

Self-assessment question answers

① By what mechanisms does the renin–angiotensin–aldosterone system act as an effector arm in the control of systemic blood pressure?

Angiotensin II acts as a direct peripheral vasoconstrictor as well as enhancing sodium chloride reabsorption in the proximal tubule, thereby acting to expand ECF volume. Aldosterone further contributes to volume expansion by stimulating sodium reabsorption in the distal nephron.

② Name some lifestyle factors which have been proven to be risk factors for the development of hypertension.

Obesity, excessive salt intake, excessive alcohol intake and physical inactivity have all been shown to be correctable lifestyle factors contributing to the development of hypertension.

③ Name three organs which are major targets for tissue damage during uncontrolled hypertension.

The brain, where cerebrovascular disease develops as a result of hypertensive effects in small and large vessels;

the heart, which is affected by left ventricular hypertrophy as well as accelerated coronary artery disease; and the kidneys, which are affected by progressive glomerular ischaemia (nephrosclerosis) with ultimate progression to chronic renal failure.

④ Why does hypertension develop when blood flow into one kidney is restricted by renal artery disease?

In the early phase of renal artery stenosis, the affected kidney becomes ischaemic, with the release of renin and subsequent activation of angiotensin II in the circulation, leading to systemic vasoconstriction. At a later phase in the disease, hypertensive nephrosclerosis develops in the unaffected kidney, overall GFR is reduced and a volume-retention pattern of hypertension supervenes.

⑤ Name five categories of antihypertensive drugs, citing a potential disadvantage or complication of therapy in each case.

Refer to Table 9.2

Chapter 10
Self-assessment case study answers

① What is the most likely explanation for his acute history of difficulty in passing urine?

The failure to pass urine for 12 h is probably caused by complete obstruction of urinary flow. The suprapubic signs suggest bladder enlargement and therefore indicate that the obstruction to urinary flow is likely to be at the level of the bladder neck or urethra. The longer history of difficulty in passing urine is typical of chronic obstruction because of prostatic enlargement.

② What is the likely explanation for the previous episode of dysuria, macroscopic haematuria and fever?

Urinary tract infection, either in his prostate (prostatitis) or above because of bacterial overgrowth occurring with urinary stasis.

③ Explain why his serum creatinine was elevated.

The chronic and then acute obstruction of urinary flow leads to high intraluminal pressures and disordered peristalsis above the level of obstruction. GFR falls as a combined result of this back-pressure, superimposed intrarenal haemodynamic changes (mediated by vasoactive hormones) and the subsequent development of renal scarring.

④ What is the best test to confirm the diagnosis?

Abdominal ultrasonography, which in this case should show an enlarged prostate, a full bladder and distension of the ureters and renal pelvis. In addition, there may be renal scarring if the obstruction has been longstanding.

⑤ What are the main principles of treatment in this situation, and why?

Relief of urinary tract obstruction using a bladder catheter and (subsequently) prostatectomy to prevent renal scarring and superimposed infection. In addition, there are likely to be fluid and electrolyte disturbances which may require immediate correction.

Self-assessment question answers

① Abnormalities of what structures can give rise to loin pain?
Spinal nerve roots, vertebral column, paraspinal and lumbar muscles, kidney capsule, renal pelvis, ureters, abdominal aorta, pancreas.

② How can the red urine occurring with haemolysis be distinguished from that occurring with haematuria?
Haem pigment is detected on urinalysis with both, but red blood cells are present on urine microscopy only with haematuria.

③ Describe the pathophysiology behind changes in renal blood flow and GFR during the first 24h after acute obstruction.
Initial vasodilatation is caused by the release of vasodilatory prostaglandins. Subsequent vasoconstriction is principally caused by the release of angiotensin II and thromboxane A_2. A fall in GFR is initially due to a rise in intraluminal pressure, and is subsequently also caused by vasoconstriction.

④ List the chemical composition of five types of renal calculi.
Calcium oxalate, calcium phosphate, uric acid, struvite, cystine.

Chapter 11
Self-assessment case study answers

① What factors indicate that this man is likely to develop gentamicin nephrotoxicity?
Gentamicin nephrotoxicity is likely to develop because a serum creatinine of 0.13mmol/L probably represents a mild–moderate reduction in renal function in a 68-year-old man. As gentamicin is entirely excreted by the kidney, a reduction in renal function causes an accumulation of drug and the main toxicity manifests as acute tubular necrosis.

② What factors should guide the prescription dosing schedule of gentamicin?
The dosage of gentamicin should be guided by trough levels of the drug. As the peak concentration of the drug correlates with efficacy and the trough level with toxicity, a small reduction in drug dose is recommended, with a significant increase in dosage interval.

③ List this patients's comorbidity and drug use which predispose him to hyperkalaemia.
Factors which predispose him to hyperkalaemia include:

- *Impaired renal function.*
- *Diabetes with the potential for impaired renal renin production and hyporeninaemic hypoaldosteronism.*
- *Concomitant use of ACE inhibitors, spironolactone and NSAIDs, all of which inhibit tubular potassium secretion by reducing aldosterone action in the kidney.*

④ Briefly indicate the mechanisms whereby drugs may result in acute renal failure.

Mechanisms of drug-induced nephrotoxicity:

- *Haemodynamic change (fall in GFR caused by reduced glomerular capillary pressure).*
- *Immune injury (interstitial nephritis).*
- *Glomerular injury.*
- *Tubular cell injury.*
- *Tubular crystallization.*
- *Multiple/uncertain.*

Self-assessment question answers

① Define the elimination half-life of a drug and explain how this may be altered in renal impairment.
The half-life of a drug is the time that it takes for the plasma concentration of the drug to halve after absorption is complete. If renal excretion is responsible for clearance of the drug, then a reduced renal clearance will prolong the half-life, and thus plasma concentrations of the drug are likely to be higher for an extended period. If the dosage schedule is not altered, then the drug will accumulate in the plasma, and drug toxicity may supervene.

② What factors determine whether a drug is excreted by the kidney?
Excretion of a drug by the kidney depends upon:

- *Filtration of the drug into the urine. In general, if a drug has a lower molecular weight and is less protein-bound, filtration is enhanced.*
- *Lipid solubility. In general, water-soluble drugs will be excreted but lipid-soluble drugs may be passively reabsorbed into the plasma.*
- *The presence of active transport processes that enhance the secretion or (less commonly) reabsorption of the compound. This is more likely to occur with anionic and cationic drugs where carrier-mediated mechanisms in the proximal tubule facilitating secretion into the tubular fluid exist.*

③ Describe the clinical and laboratory findings that differentiate an interstitial nephritis from a haemodynamically mediated reduction in renal function.
Interstitial nephritis is often characterized by systemic features of rash and, occasionally, arthralgia and lymphadenopathy. Peripheral blood examination often shows an eosinophilia and an elevated erythrocyte sedimentation rate. Urinalysis often reveals haematuria and proteinuria, and blood pressure is often elevated. As the diagnosis may be confused with a systemic vasculitis, it is often made on renal biopsy. In contrast, haemodynamic injury is characterized by hypotension and other features of tissue ischaemia such as mild abnormalities in liver function. Urinalysis and urine microscopy are unremarkable and clinical and laboratory features of systemic inflammation are absent. It general, it occurs in closer temporal relation to the introduction of a drug than does an interstitial nephritis and responds more quickly to withdrawal of the drug.

Appendix: normal ranges

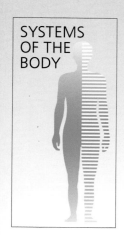

SYSTEMS
OF THE
BODY

The ranges shown are for adults unless otherwise stated.

	Range	Units
Haematology		
Haemoglobin (men)	130–180	g/L
(women)	115–165	g/L
White cell count	4.0–11.0	$\times 10^9$/L
Platelet count	150–400	$\times 10^9$/L
Packed cell volume (haematocrit)	0.38–0.52	
Erythrocyte sedimentation rate	3–15	mm/h
Biochemistry		
Venous plasma or serum		
Sodium (Na)	135–145	mmol/L
Potassium (K)	3.5–5.0	mmol/L
Chloride (Cl)	95–110	mmol/L
Bicarbonate (HCO_3^- or 'total CO_2')	22–30	mmol/L
Urea	3.0–8.0	mmol/L
Creatinine (adults)	0.06–0.12	mmol/L
(children)	0.03–0.08	mmol/L
Osmolality	280–300	mosm/kg water
Glucose ('BSL') (fasting)	3.0–5.4	mmol/L
(random)	3.0–7.7	mmol/L
HbA_{1C}	3.5–6.0	%
Total protein	62–80	g/L
Albumin	32–45	g/L
Total calcium (Ca)	2.10–2.60	mmol/L
Phosphate (PO_4)	0.8–1.5	mmol/L
Magnesium (Mg)	0.8–1.0	mmol/L
Urate	0.2–0.4	mmol/L
Total cholesterol	< 5.5	mmol/L
Triglycerides (fasting)	< 2.0	mmol/L
Arterial blood		
pO_2	80–105	mmHg
pCO_2	35–45	mmHg
pH	7.36–7.44	
HCO_3^-	22–30	mmol/L
Urine		
Protein	< 150	mg/24 h
Urate	2.0–6.6	mmol/24 h
Calcium	2.5–7.5	mmol/24 h
Creatinine (depends on muscle mass)	6–16	mmol/24 h
Sodium (depends on intake)	50–200	mmol/24 h
Potassium (depends on intake)	40–100	mmol/24 h
Osmolality (depends on hydration)	50–1200	mosm/kg water

Immunology

Antinuclear antibodies (ANA)	1 : 100 or less	
dsDNA antibodies	< 7	IU/mL
Complement:		
C3	0.75–1.75	g/L
C4	0.10–0.40	g/L

Microbiology

Midstream urine – microscopy and culture

White blood cells	< 10	$\times 10^6$/L
Red blood cells	< 10	$\times 10^6$/L
Epithelial cells	< 10	$\times 10^6$/L
Bacterial colony count	< 10^7	/L

GLOSSARY

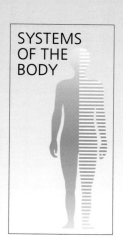

SYSTEMS
OF THE
BODY

adrenocortical hormones – steroid hormones produced by the adrenal cortex, including cortisol and aldosterone.

amyloidosis – a systemic disease in which a waxy, starch-like glycoprotein (amyloid) accumulates in tissues and organs.

anorexia – loss of appetite.

antinuclear antibodies – auto-antibodies which react with nuclear material.

arterio-venous nipping – narrowing of the venules in the retina at the point where they are crossed by arterioles, seen on fundoscopy of the eye in states of hypertension.

arteriopathy – any pathological condition affecting the arteries.

asterixis – a coarse flapping tremor seen in the limbs during severe metabolic disturbances.

atherosclerosis – a degenerative disease affecting arteries, characterised by deposition of lipid plaques in the inner layers of the walls of medium and large sized arteries.

atrial fibrillation – a cardiac arrhythmia characterised by disorganised electrical activity in the atria accompanied by a rapid, irregular ventricular response.

auscultation – the process of listening for sounds within body organs (especially the heart and lungs) to assess normality or signs of disease.

bipolar affective disorder – a psychiatric condition characterised by episodes of excitement, depression, or mixed mood, usually associated at some time with delusions or other major thought disorder.

bruit – an abnormal sound or murmur heard while auscultating over a blood vessel or organ.

cirrhosis – chronic liver disease involving fibrosis (scarring) and nodular regeneration.

claudication – cramp-like pains felt typically in the calves during walking, caused by inadequate arterial circulation.

complement – a series of enzymatic serum proteins involved in mediating the inflammatory consequences of antigen-antibody reactions.

crepitations (crackles) – crackling noise heard during auscultation of the lung in conditions involving fluid exudation into the alveolar airspaces.

dialysis – procedure for altering the chemical composition of the blood, particularly in renal failure, involving the diffusion of solutes through a semi-permeable membrane, either externally (in the case of haemodialysis), or internally (in the case of peritoneal dialysis).

differential diagnosis – the consideration of a number of alternative diseases as the cause for a patient's presentation.

diverticular disease – a condition of the colon involving the development of pouch-like herniations through the muscular layer of the bowel wall, prone to local rupture resulting in inflammation and abscess formation (diverticulitis).

DMSA – dimercaptosuccinic acid, a chemical used for radionuclide studies of the integrity of the renal parenchyma.

DTPA – diethylene triamine penta-acetic acid, a chemical used for radionuclide studies of organ function, particularly blood flow through the kidney.

end-stage renal failure – chronic renal failure (reduction in glomerular filtration rate) so advanced as to be incompatible with life without the institution of a form of renal replacement therapy (dialysis or transplantation).

fenestrated – (of a membrane) characterised by the presence of numerous small holes or openings.

glomerulopathy – any pathological condition affecting the glomeruli of the kidney.

glycoside – a chemical often of plant origin that yields a sugar and a non sugar on hydrolysis (e.g. digitalis).

glycosuria – the presence of glucose in the urine.

Goodpasture's syndrome – an inflammatory condition involving the lungs (causing pulmonary bleeding) and the kidneys (causing glomerulonephritis), characterised by autoimmune antibody formation to basement membrane antigens.

habitus (bodily) – the overall bodily appearance or physique.

hyperglobulinaemia (polyclonal) – an increase in the concentration of globulin proteins in the plasma (these having different antigenic specificities).

metastatic calcification – deposition of calcium salts in previously healthy soft tissues.

microscopic polyangiitis (polyarteritis) – an inflammatory condition of the walls of small-sized arteries, producing focal ischaemia in the affected tissues.

myeloma (multiple) – a plasma cell tumour arising in the bone marrow (in multiple sites).

osteitis fibrosa cystica – pathological changes of bone in severe hyperparathyroidism, involving replacement of normal bone by cysts and fibrous tissue.

osteomalacia – a condition of reduced calcification of the matrix of lamellar bone, resulting in bone weakness and predisposition to fracture.

osteoporosis – a condition of reduced bone density, occurring most frequently in post menopausal women and in catabolic states.

papillary necrosis – death of the renal papillae, the innermost segment of the medullary pyramids.

paraprotein – an immunoglobulin of a single type, over-produced during a plasma cell disorder.

parenchyma – the specialised tissue of a particular organ (e.g. kidney).

parenteral alimentation – provision of nutritional requirements by a route other than the digestive tract (typically intravenously).

pericarditis – inflammation of the pericardial sac surrounding the heart.

rigor – an episode of coarse shivering that may be associated with chills and fever.

stent – a cylindrical device made of artificial material used to maintain the patency of a vessel or tubular structure in the body.

syndrome – a combination of symptoms (complaints) and signs (physical features), which characterise a particular disease or inherited condition.

systemic lupus erythematosus (SLE) – an autoimmune inflammatory disorder affecting multiple body systems.

thrombocytopenia – an abnormally low platelet count in the blood.

tubulo-interstitium – the component of the kidney parenchyma consisting of the tubules and the interstitial tissue.

tumour lysis syndrome – condition resulting from the rapid breakdown of malignant tissue, typically after chemotherapy.

uraemia (uraemic syndrome) – a biochemical and clinical state associated with the presence of large amounts of urea and other nitrogenous waste products in the blood, as occurs in advanced renal failure.

urinalysis – a chemical examination of the urine, most commonly performed using a dipstick containing reagents impregnated on paper squares.

INDEX

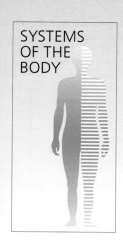

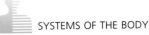